I0082712

1

Fasting and Intermittent Fasting Diet Bundle for Quick and Healthy Weight Loss

Fasting and Intermittent Fasting Diet Bundle for Quick and Healthy Weight Loss

Includes Intermittent Fasting for Weight loss, an Intermittent Fasting Meal Plan, and The Complete Guide to Fasting

Kyle Faber

Fasting and Intermittent Fasting Diet Bundle for Quick and Healthy Weight Loss

Includes Intermittent Fasting for Weight Loss, an Intermittent Fasting Meal Plan, and the Complete Guide to Fasting

Copyright © 2018 Kyle Faber

All rights reserved. No portion of this book may be reproduced, stored in a retrieval system, or transmitted in any form or by any means – electronic, mechanical, photocopy, recording, scanning, or other – except for brief quotations in critical reviews or articles, without prior written permission of the publisher.

Published by CAC Publishing LLC.

ISBN 978-1-948489-99-7 paperback

ISBN 978-1-948489-98-0 eBook

The Fasting Book:
The Complete Guide to Unlocking the Miracle of Fasting

Healing the Body, Sharpening the Mind, Energizing the Spirit

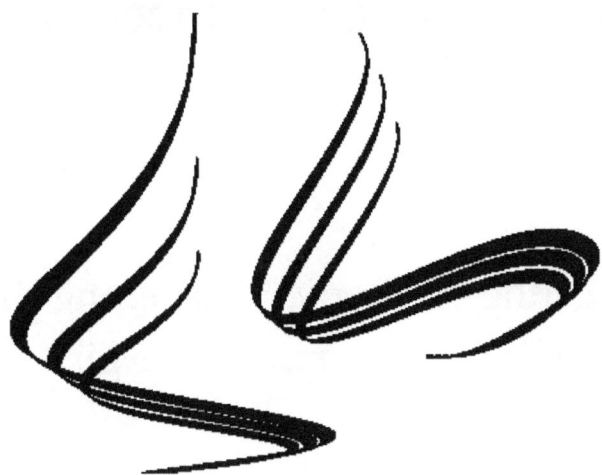

The Fasting Book:

The Complete Guide to Unlocking the Miracle of Fasting

Healing the Body, Sharpening the Mind, Energizing the Spirit

Kyle Faber

Copyright © 2017 by Kyle Faber

All rights reserved. No part of this publication may be reproduced, distributed, or transmitted in any form or by any means, including photocopying, recording, or other electronic or mechanical methods, without the prior written permission of the publisher, except in the case of brief quotations embodied in critical reviews and certain other noncommercial uses permitted by copyright law.

CAC Publishing LLC

ISBN: 978-1-948489-22-5 paperback

ISBN: 978-1-948489-21-8 eBook

This book is dedicated to those that wish to embark on the journey to fasting and clarity. To those that wish to heal their bodies, sharpen their minds, and reenergize their spirits. May you find what you are in search of and let it be all you hoped it would be.

Preface

"I think that the Dr. Tanners and those others who go forty days without eating do it by resolutely keeping out the desire to eat, in the beginning, and that after a few hours the desire is discouraged and comes no more"

Mark Twain

Paleontologists agree that the genetic makeup that dominates our current state was set sometime back around 50,000 BCE in the late Paleolithic. Our ancestors of that era survived as hunter-gatherers foraging for food they could find and hunting for animals they had to chase down. The task of finding and hunting meant that food was not always available. When they managed to hunt, it was time to feast. When they had none, the famine could last for days. That feast and fast cycle was the norm back then. While they didn't eat anything they still had to muster the energy to hunt or gather their source of energy.

That essentially meant two things.

First, humans had to expend energy in the act of foraging or hunting for food.

Second, they went through cycles of feast and fast. The body had to adapt to the reality of the day which was to be able to take in lots of food and store it for later use when there was no food to be found.

The process of evolution and natural selection basically set our body types to thrive in these conditions and our genetic structure has pretty much stayed the same all this time since then.

Fast forward 50 millennia and the problem is that our ability to organize ourselves advanced faster than our body has been able to evolve and adapt.

Civilizations, technology, and economics have allowed for the efficient distribution of labor and resources which have resulted in the abundance of food. In today's world, we are presented with this abundance of food and a relatively sedentary lifestyle.

Both these factors result in a mismatch between our existing energy storage and utilization patterns inherent in our system and our current practices. This results in extended weight gain, reduction in efficiency, chronic illnesses and even fatality.

Our bodies that were designed to accumulate energy stores and serve them up during periods of famine don't have the opportunity these days to go hungry and burn up the excess stores. Instead, we keep gaining the weight. That has a detrimental effect on our body, our mind and in the end what we think of as security and progress is actually what's killing us and robbing us of our potential.

We all have some kinds of perception of fasting. That's normal human behavior. But fasting is much more than just the cessation of food intake. It's about getting to know the different parts of your mind, the various mindsets you harbor and the motivations behind your actions and behavior.

Fasting is a powerful act that binds the body, mind, and spirit in a way that empowers you. If you just want to lose the extra weight, then yes, fasting will help, but you should use fasting as a way to change your life and improve your fortunes.

If you want to look and feel younger, fasting has proven to do that because it is able to activate the growth hormones that aesthetic doctors charge a bomb just to administer hormones like the HGH.

Fasting is not an option. It is a necessity when you understand the body and what it is designed to do. It is also an amazing source of power when you realize that if you alter the environment your body is subjected to and move with the natural rhythm of your energy management cycles, you will find that you get healthier, which means you probably live longer. You will find, as I have, that you are able to think better, which means you will do better in life. If you can sort out the chaos between the mind and the body, you will find that you have better access to your inner peace – the soul within.

This book is about fasting – revealing the reasons you should fast, the benefits you get from fasting and how to do it correctly for optimal results. We are going to take you on a trip and show you exactly what your body, mind, and spirit have been doing in the absence of fasting, and what it can do once you make fasting a part of your life.

This book is not about fad diets. It's not about serious diets like the Atkins, or the Paleo diet. It's not seasonal and it's not expensive. Everything you need is here, in this book; and within you.

Shedding the pounds, increasing your vitality and extending your lifespan, are just a few things you can achieve, but there is more. A lot more.

Fasting is the secret act that some of the most successful people do in the privacy of their own thought. They may tell you about their meditation, they may tell you about all the hard work they put in. They may even tell you about the laws of attraction and how they went all out to make it. But the one thing that successful people don't tell you is the hard core fasting that they do.

Fasting will change your life on the inside as much as it changes your look on the outside. Fasting will sharpen your focus and increase your ability to think preemptively thereby doing more than anything else you can ever do.

With fasting, there is no short cut. You have to feel the discomfort and come out the other side. You have to feel the despair and the pain that you will at the height of your fast and yet find the will to push through. When you come out the other side, you will be a brand new person. You will look better, your skin will radiate better. You will even walk better. You will sleep better and you will see life better as well.

Fasting is the secret and the miracle you need to change your life - and you control it.

It is the act of fasting that takes you from being a spectator to being a contender. It is fasting that will take you from being sluggish and out of shape to being sharp and highly effective. Fasting results in more than just a better figure - it also shapes the mind. Fasting mindfully and consistently will change your life and your lifespan.

We have begun to awaken as a species. We have begun to understand the world around us, we understand better every day how to wade through the noise and latch on to what is real and what is beneficial in the long term. What we've known for over two thousand years is that fasting has an almost miraculous effect on the body and the mind. When you improve the body and the mind, you empower your spirit, and that makes all the difference.

The human experience is influenced by internal forces and the external environment. Free will, discipline, and imagination gives us the ability to alter the sum of these forces and navigate our trajectory through an unpredictable environment.

We are exceptional beings - the result of millions of iterations in a long chain of evolutionary links. No doubt we are still a work in progress, but our power is beyond that of any other creature in existence.

That power comes in many forms, but what it results in is ultimately the empowering of each person who is willing to put in the effort and endure the discomfort to get across to the greatness within them.

This greatness does not come from our apparent ability to lord over the animal and plant kingdoms of the world, explore the depths of the planet or launch ourselves into the farthest reaches of space. No. Our greatness comes, instead, from our ability to convert the intangible into reality. That is not a small feat, and you have the ability to do it. All you need is the power of your spirit to be able to tap into the universe of inspiration and a mind that is resilient and un-enslaved to anyone or anything.

The human condition is one that should never cease to amaze you. Look at all the things we have accomplished and that will amaze you, I am sure. But if you pause for a moment and consider all the things that haven't been done and realize that we are capable of even that, that's the point that you will be blown away.

Introduction

The key to life is balance. But the noun in this context should not be attached to the equal distribution of opposing states. You can't think that you need an equal amount of positive experiences in life with an equal amount of negative ones. You can't think that you need to be happy 50% of the time and sad the remaining 50. And, in the name of balance, you shouldn't be gyrating between the indulgence and austerity.

Fasting is about balance. But instead of it being, as you may think, the source of balance, it's not. Fasting is about returning the balance between the forces of your being - the mind, body, and spirit.

The balance we seek in the well of fasting is ultimately a delicate one that we hope to strike on a daily basis, but it's not always possible to achieve. That balance is one that is unique to each of us and can't really be compared. The point of balance between the three forces that I am driven by is slightly different from what you will be driven by. There really isn't a quantitative measure that we can describe it with either. It would be foolish to try and describe how much each person needs to put in, and so the measure of our perfect state is defined by the overall outcome of our efforts.

It took years for me to find my unique state in which I am able to achieve my best. There were numerous attempts and failures, some attempts and partial successes and finally the right balance was achieved. I suspect it is designed this way (I use the term 'design' freely) because in the midst of finding that balance I found who I am and what balance of mind, body, and spirit, I need to bring to the table to beat the bank.

Chapter 1 Metabolic Profiles

Your ideal state is one of balance between the forces that bear on your existence. These forces are a function of a number of factors and when it comes to physicality and physiology, the forces that weigh on you depend on your metabolic profile.

It helps to narrow things down based on your general frame that describes your inherent - metabolic profile. Nothing in this world is one-size-fits-all - even fasting.

There are three main metabolic, and you will fall into one of them: the slow metabolic profile; mild metabolic profile; and, the fast metabolic profile. Don't let the names hang you up it's just for reference it doesn't mean that you're slow or fast, it just relates to how quickly you burn energy for a given state.

As the description of the three natural metabolic profiles takes shape you will come across the notion of being in or out of balance. There isn't a net disadvantage of being in one or the other profiles. But it would be suboptimal for any profile type to be out of balance.

The notion of being in or out of balance is something that you will slowly come to know as you explore how your body, mind, and spirit behave in theoretical isolation and excel in practical union.

The balance you seek is characterized by the state where the three elements of your being come together in the right formula and result in great power, able to make the best of your existence. It is the deep sense of motivation that makes conquerors conquer, athletes inspire, performers dazzle, and the human race accomplish feats that bewilder the uninspired.

The three metabolic profiles are described below and help you ascertain your body type so that when it comes to fasting and energy, you will know what to expect moving forward. It is especially important to know your profile so that you know the best way to prepare for the fast.

Slow Metabolic Profile

If your metabolic profile is slow, you are characterized by a larger and more solid frame. You will be overweight if you are out of balance, but you are strong when you are in balance. You will also have tremendous stamina and be able to endure heavy activity for long periods of time. You will not necessarily be overweight if you are balanced, but a lot of what you carry beyond your ideal weight will be water weight, and you will not have a typically muscular silhouette even if they are present.

You are the kind that will normally feel relaxed and find it hard to get your energy up or get excited. There is a purpose to this, and when you take advantage of your inherent strength you will find that you can achieve a lot over the long haul.

But when you are imbalanced, when you put on the weight, when you consume high quantities of sugar and take in excess food, you start to gain weight easily. Sugar and caffeine are especially appealing to you because they seem to give you the boost of energy that you enjoy. This is when you go out of balance and the time when you need to turn to fasting to bring everything back in check.

From a mental perspective, you have strong memory and are able to think through things strategically. When you are out of balance, you are easily driven towards mild depression and are easily distracted.

You are suited to longer periods of fasting. If you are on a total water fast, and you are used to shorter fasts, then you have it in you to take it to 30 days and feel the power of it all.

To get a visual of what it means to have a slow metabolic profile think of these following people: Catherine Zeta-Jones, Jennifer Lopez, Angelina Jolie, Nigella Lawson, Queen Latifah, Liv Tyler, Beyoncé, Oprah Winfrey, Antonio Banderas, Shaquille O'Neal, Placido Domingo, Tom Hanks, Harrison Ford, and Kevin Kline.

Mild Metabolic Profile

People of mild metabolic constitutions are generally tall, and slender when they are in balance. They are generally quick to absorb information, but also quick to forget. If this is you, then you are generally intelligent, athletic, and outgoing. When you are out of balance you tend to indulge in negative thoughts and are prone to long periods of deep depression. When you are in balance, you can move the world with your charm and your will power alone.

Food is your ally when taken in moderation, and when out of balance your fasting needs to be less rigorous than the one someone of a slow metabolic profile requires. You should take your fasting slow. Doing 24-hour fasts. Then once you get used to it, do 72-hour fasts and work your way up to a week. Don't rush it if you are in this metabolic profile.

You have tons of energy that are ideally suited to be applied in short bursts, unlike the long distance stamina people in the last category display.

Generally, people in this category have similar frames and disposition of the following people: Cameron Diaz, Nicole Kidman, Uma Thurman, Penelope Cruz, Kate Hudson, Halle Berry, Jennifer Garner, Keira Knightley, Courteney Cox, Gwyneth Paltrow, Jim Carrey, Noah Wyle, Prince William, Ben Affleck, David Duchovny, Will Smith, Ashton Kutcher, and Orlando Bloom.

Rapid Metabolic Profile

Those with rapid profiles are characterized by people who are generally slim, tall, and athletic; and are super-fast at whatever they tend to be interested in. They are also highly strung if they are out of balance and tend to have skin problems. People in this category make record breaking athletes and are the body type that needs tremendous amounts of discipline to be able to reach their balance and excel in their chosen career.

These types also tend to get hungry often, they tend to snack a lot, the love sugar because they have seen in the past that sugar gives them the energy that they constantly crave for. But the sugar they need to take is typically from sweet fruits like bananas and not the raw, processed sugar that they find in the grocery store.

To get an idea of what this profile looks like take a look at the following people: Sharon Stone, Debra Messing, Britney Spears, Jennifer Aniston, Hilary Duff, Mia Hamm, Brad Pitt, Tom Cruise, Justin Timberlake, Denzel Washington, Kobe Bryant, and Lance Armstrong.

People in this category should think seriously if they are planning on fasting. There really isn't much need and you should start with 12 – 18-hour fasts. You need to drink lots of water on regular non-fasting days, and even more water on fasting days. The reason you do not fast for too long is that you are probably at your ideal weight or lower. If you are above your ideal weight, stick to 3-day fasts or less. Then return to regular eating, and then back to your diet again.

For all three types remember that you are not in this for some Olympic Fasting medal. You are here to reach an objective. That objective is to have a healthy body support a strong mind so that you can gain the power of an energized spirit.

Chapter One Take Away
Here is what you need to take away from this chapter. Figure out your profile based on some of the characteristics mentioned in this chapter and

confirm that by looking at the people who are in those profiles. Figuring out your metabolic profile is not rocket science and is fairly easy to do. This is your first step and an important one since it determines the kind of fasting you should do.

***

Chapter 2 Balance

The balance is not achieved by gluttony one day and total fasting the next. The balance and harmony you need to supercharge your life comes from balance that is accomplished using small variations.

The typical human body can take about 40 days of total fasting. Some can do 50 under perfect conditions. And in that time, the body can do miraculous things, but not all of us need to resort to those sorts of extremes for a prolonged basis.

The purpose of fasting is not to lose weight but to get healthy in body, mind, and spirit. Fasting is the one path that you can take to understand yourself and change your life at the same time. Fasting is the only thing that can get you back in balance regardless of which metabolic type you are.

Fasting is not meant to be carried out every day for the long haul. It is meant as a balancing tool. Whenever you are out of balance, use fasting as a means of returning.

There are many kinds of fasting programs that you will come across. There is the water fast, the Biblical fast, the one-day fast, the seven-day fast. The juice fast. You name it, it's out there.

But before you even take one step toward any kind of fasting, you need to pause and understand what you are in search of. For me, it was instinctual. I wanted to clear the toxins coursing through my body and shooting through my mind. For me, transformation was the result of a slow process of conversion from foodie to 'fastie'. To fast, you need to change your mind, not your stomach. You need to reset your mindset, not adjust your diet.

States of Body and States of Mind

When you look at the body and the mind, there are just so many factors to consider. To make it simple, look at your body and your mind as a function of states. Your state of mind and your state of body are inextricably linked. If you want to change one, change the other and watch the effect.

You know what your state of mind can be like. You get happy, you get moody, you get inspired, and so on. There are many states of mind that you can think of but for now, take that concept of states and apply it to your body, and there are few that you should concern yourself with. There is the state of fasting (since we are a book on fasting). The second is a state of digesting. The third is a stage of activity. The forth is a state of rest.

You can combine two of those states: Fasting and activity, digesting and rest, fasting and rest, and digesting and activity.

There is no such thing as the best state or the worst pair among these four. They all serve a different net function. What you need to do is to be able to consciously find the best pair of states and balance it through your day.

Each of us have different balancing points; your goal is to find that point of balance. A typical point of balance would be to have x amount of time in the Fasting and Active state, x1 amount of time in the Fasting and Rest state, y amount of time in the Digesting and Active state and y1 time in the Digestive and Rest state. Your total daily clock is 24 hours and with the proper balance of these four states, you can even be productive while you sleep.

Balance of Energy

Another thing you need to realize is that the body has two sources of energy. The first is the energy that comes directly from the food that you consume and directly absorbed into your blood stream.

Whatever energy you use during the day for respiration and activity, is burnt up, but whatever you don't use remains in the system – it's a simple concept that we all know about. The excess is stored in a way that the body can use whenever it needs to. It is stored within the body for future use. The energy that is stored for future use is stored in the form of adipose tissue and is what results in gaining weight. We call this fat.

Fat is a form of energy. It's not a bad thing in general terms. Fat is the energy we stored when we ate more than our body needed to power itself. As our Paleo ancestors did some 50,000 years ago, we too are storing food for later use in case of famine.

It is how we adapted to irregular food supply schedules – as we talked about earlier. That history gives us a clue into our point of balance. We realize that our bodies don't gain weight because it's flawed. We realize we gain weight because of our environment and the way we adapted to it.

But the problem is that our lifestyle and practices have changed so far beyond the tolerances that we are feeding our bodies more food than it needs and working it less than we should. That accumulates over the years and it alters our state of mind, state of physicality and defines us through the problems those imbalances cause us.

What's the problem?

Well, there are two problems with this and that requires two answers. The first problem is that we have gone out of balance and we need to get back to it. The second problem is that we need to find a way to stay in balance, or at least a way where we don't stray so far from it that illnesses and degenerative diseases start to dictate and define us.

The first problem of how to return to balance is easy – you already know it instinctively. That is too fast. When you fast, as you are coming to realize, all those excess stores are utilized and the body can return to its state of balance.

The second issue is to not stray too far from that balance, and to do that we need a lifestyle change – a new point of balance, where the accumulation is less but we still stay in touch with the methods of our times.

The solution is to fast according to your metabolic profile, and then change your daily energy management plan which includes more physically strenuous activity and lesser total food consumption per day.

That takes care of the genetic pattern that we are endowed with. But something else has taken over our lifestyle choices and that is habit. Habit is wholly located within the realm of the mind.

Because we are trained to segment our day and sit down to three square meals, it has become habitual and expected of us. Our social traps even revolve around this habit and it has become so ingrained in us that it has pushed our point of balance even further to the fringe of our design limits. Changing those habits requires a new set of practices to break the old habits, then consciously instill a new set of practices and allow them to take root as habits.

This takes time and the consequences can be harsh. Eating is a habit, and eating throughout the day is a widespread habit. There is a price to be paid to change this habit and that price is the development of your will. The way to build that is by fasting as well.

Chapter Two Take Away

Fasting is a tool that moves you to a new balance. Think of it as a lever that moves you from your complacent point of balance now to a healthier point of balance – one that takes your natural genetic design and applies it to current conveniences.

You can come back and use this tool whenever you want, whether it's to balance your physical self or to rebalance your mind. Both work. Remember fasting is the tool that moves your balance, to stay there you need a lifestyle change.

***

Chapter 3 Things to Know

Before we jump in and get fasting, you should fully understand a few things that pertain to your physiology and how we all react to food and the environment around us. There are a number of misconceptions that we have taken to be true.

There are people out there, I have come across, who, until today, can't tell the functional difference between nutrition and calories, or the difference between appetite and hunger.

These are explained in this chapter and along with some of the other tools you need to arm yourself with as you undertake this path to reach your powerful balance.

Calories vs. Nutrients

We will start with nutrition and calories. Calories measure the units of energy your body needs. Your body uses energy for all kinds of things. Without energy, you couldn't climb the stairs or blink your eyelids. Energy is the fuel you need to perform every task from thinking to digesting.

How much is one calorie? Well to help you conceptualize it just think of it this way – a calorie is the amount of energy it takes to raise the temperature of one gram of water by one degree Celsius. For practical purposes when it comes to food, we measure it in kcal – kilocalories which is the measure of change of 1000 grams of water by 1 degree Celsius.

Energy is typically gained from sugars, but that doesn't mean that's the only source. Everything you consume can be converted to energy, even if you squash up a piece of paper, once digested there are calories in it. We typically get our calories, or at least the bulk of it, from carbohydrates.

Nutrients, on the other hand, are different from calories. Nutrients include all the vitamins and minerals that your body needs to make enzymes, tissue, bone, muscle, neurons, and every other part of you, inside and out. Some nutrients are important to the proper functioning of the body but cannot be synthesized by the body and are thus taken in by ingestion. These are the building blocks of the human body and are used to repair the parts of you that deplete on a daily basis due to wear and tear.

For instance, you need iron so that your blood can carry oxygen. Iron can't be synthesized by the body and needs to be consumed from external sources. You already have iron in your blood and marrows, but as you replace old hemoglobin cells with new ones, the old ones are processed and flushed out of your system. You replace the ones that are flushed out by taking in new iron from various sources in your diet.

What you have to think about when you consider fasting is not just how your body is constantly kept energized, it's also about how your body is kept in optimal shape by taking in the nutrients it needs when it needs it.

Fasting plays a huge role in this process because it hones your ability to understand what your body needs and not what your brain may misinterpret from the signals coming from the body.

Fasting puts you in better health because it allows your systems to get the right balance of calories and nutrients. It also allows you to shed the excess calories that you have inadvertently taken in due to your need for nutrients.

When you feel hungry, your body is in need of one, or both, of two things. It either needs calories to sustain its activities, or it needs nutrients for its upkeep process. In the event you eat a meal that has the calories but not the nutrients, your body is going to continue to send messages to the brain that it needs food to satisfy the nutrient needs.

So for instance, if you are in need of iron, but your meal is void of any iron content, you will have loaded up on calories (and other nutrients) and satisfied the need for energy, but you would have taken none of the iron that the body needed. So a little while after you've had your meal and the body found no iron in what you consumed, you will feel hungry again. Hunger is not always a call for energy, it can be, and many times it is, a call for nutrients. And in the world of processed foods, much of what is available to us along the aisles of supermarkets are foods stripped of their nutrients and repackaged in a way that creates addictions rather than supplying nutrients.

Most people load up when they feel hungry thinking that they need the calories, but they fail to realize that it's the nutrients that the body needs that they are missing.

But how do you know what the body is asking for - nutrients, calories, or both? That's where fasting comes in. When you fast, it changes your physiology to the point that you will effectively start to understand the signals your body sends you on what it needs. And if you get into the discipline of balancing your meals with high nutrient-content foods and low-calorie processed-food contents, you will start to have better ratios in calories to nutrients.

Here are foods with high-nutrient/low-calorie ratios:

a.   Salmon
b.   Sardines

c.   Kale
d.   Garlic
e.   Seaweed
f.   Clams
g.   Oysters
h.   Beef (focus on the liver)
i.   Blueberries
j.   Cocoa (85% Dark Chocolate)

High Caloric Intake

This is a problem with society in general today, we take in so many empty calories and that seems to have bloated the average weight of the entire nation. We are more than 20 pounds overweight on average here in the United States and that is still not painting the proper picture. The effects of obesity include Type 2 Diabetes and various cardiac issues, not to mention secondary issues arising from poorly performing organs that are clogged up with fat tissue.

Because each of us falls into a different metabolic group as described earlier, it's hard to put a pin in exactly what your caloric intake should be on a daily basis. But on average, it is accepted that men have a higher caloric burn rate than women and, as such, men are given an allowance of about 1800 calories per day, while women are said to need about 1200 calories per day.

This will vary according to your lifestyle.

If you do a one-hour heavy calorie-burn workout every morning, it is more likely that you will burn more during the course of the day. If you roll out of bed and sit on your bean bag to telecommute to work then you are going to have a much lower caloric burn rate through your day.

It also matters when and how you work out. Since we don't know what our caloric burn rate is, I for one believe it's pointless to count calories and instead focus on how you eat and when you eat.

There are two things you need to understand when it comes to calories because not all calories are created equal. They have different profiles. Calories from items with high glycemic values have a detrimental effect compared to one with a low glycemic index.

Our high caloric intake can be attributed to high intake of highly processed foods and we do that as a force of habit and a form of addiction.

We take in large quantities of empty calories because we do not heed our real appetites but instead pay attention to hunger and the pleasurable feedback of fulfilled habits derived from eating. If you can understand the concept of appetite and differentiate hunger from appetite, and then further distinguish those from just being greedy, then you would have come a long way in eating healthy.

Distinguishing, hunger, appetite, and greed, is exactly what fasting will end up teaching you and allow you to be able to take control of your choice of intake and your ability to lead a balanced and healthy life. Most of the sensations you feel as hunger are actually triggered by habit and by greed - the desire to taste food in your mouth.

Appetite vs. Hunger

You need to get a clear understanding of appetite and you need to be able to understand the difference between appetite and hunger. Have you ever been ill and not had the appetite to eat? Sure you have. You've even had the sensation of being hungry but not had the appetite to eat anything.

When you don't have the appetite, it is the part of you that knows it shouldn't be eating or the part of you that doesn't need any nutrients - you just need the calories or it's just habit kicking in. Even animals have the same instinct. When dogs are sick, they curl up and stay away from food. Why? Because fasting the body gives it a chance to heal itself. So even though you feel hungry, you don't have the appetite.

Hunger is the feeling you get when your body is looking for calories or nutrition. On the other hand, appetite is the body making a choice of what it wants to eat. When you say that "Hey, I am in the mood for Salmon, there is a good chance that your body is looking for Omega 3 (or something that the body needs and knows it can get if you chose salmon)." If you listen closely, your body will tell you what you need to feed it in order for the body to get what it needs. That's what appetites are for.

The body is a simple mechanism; it sends unambiguous messages to the brain on what it needs. The problem arises when the brain interprets what the body needs. If the brain misinterprets the appetite sensation from the body, then the body ends up getting what it didn't ask for. In this situation, the body then goes on to ask for it again, and you end up feeling hungry.

The typical response to hunger is to find food, regardless of what you feel like eating. If you get the message right and you give the body what it's looking for, what happens is that it satisfies the hunger, and the body moves on.

There are some things that the body needs in large quantities, and there are some things it needs in smaller quantities, so the ones that it doesn't need too much of, you won't get the appetite for it so often. For instance, if you are well into a muscle building program at the gym and you are using up large amounts of protein, your body is going to have the appetite for protein rich foods — whatever that may be in your corner of the world. If you are used to eating meat, your body will have the appetite for steak, for instance. If you are vegetarian, you may feel the cravings of eating soy burgers.

This is the reason pregnant moms get strange cravings. The body is in the process of building a whole new body inside and it needs all kinds of building blocks that it needs to get from different kinds of food. So the craving is just a more intense kind of appetite - a way for you to get a particular nutrient the body needs.

How does fasting alter or affect this?

This is where it gets interesting. The body has three concurrent systems that are at play. There is the actual body that creates a craving for a particular nutrient by association. It doesn't tell you it needs Vitamin C, you just get the urge to drink orange juice. It doesn't tell you it needs phosphorus, you just feel like having chocolate. But how does your body know what to ask for? It doesn't. It learns.

A good way to understand this is to observe how you feel thirsty. When the body starts to lose water and parts of the body goes dry, you feel a sensation of dryness in your throat, and that's the feeling, but it's your brain that interprets that feeling and deduces you are thirsty prompting you to take action.

The first few times you drink, let's say, orange juice as a kid, your body records all the things it can get from orange juice. The first time you have a burger it records all the things you get from that burger. The first time you have something sweet, it records the sudden burst of energy, and it realizes how much energy sugar has, and you start to like sugar more often.

But in today's crazy world of fast food, processed foods, and engineered foods, the body is tricked into liking certain kinds of foods. Scientists have found that the body gets hooked on a particular combination of salt, sugar, and fats. If you design a product with the right ratio, you will hook the customer for life and alter their tastes. Power drink manufacturers rely on this too and inject drinks with sugar and caffeine. These two products are targeted to teenagers and the result twenty years later is an entire generation that has a problem choosing the right food. What you end up with is a body that is constantly hungry from not getting the nutrients it needs, but too many calories from the engineered foods. The result: an overweight population.

The second system is the part of the brain that receives the impulses from the body with the raw information that the body is in need of nutrition and energy. This part of the brain is fairly primal and all it knows to do is to equate the impulses from the body and translate them. In the case of the changes in the body's chemistry, the brain detects the changes and determines that it needs to acquire food.

The third system is the conscious mind that looks at this sensation from the primal brain and decides if it's is time to eat or if there are other pressing matters to attend to. In the event that it is not an opportune moment to stop for a meal, the notion to stop for a meal is cast aside. It is also this part of the brain that interprets the appetite and cravings.

These are the three parts that go into the hunger and meal acquisition process.

Habits

We all have habits. We have morning habits, we have sleeping habits, even our walking, and gait, is a habit. Habits have three elements to it. There is an event, that event triggers a desire, and at the point of satisfaction of that desire, there is a reward. There is a negative version of that as well. If there is a desire but it's not fulfilled, there is a pain in response.

In the case of eating, there is a habit function as well. The body is designed to eat at a certain time based on social norms. Just like Pavlov's dogs that salivate at the sound of a bell, we humans salivate at the chime of a clock. This is not real hunger, this is habit.

What you feel as hunger, most of the time, is a habit that is trying to get you to do something that you don't need.

Fear

Another primitive part of you is the emotion of fear. We say primitive because this part of you is binary and it can be traced back to as far as the start of land based creatures. When the first creatures evolved from plant life, the defining factors that shaped evolution was the mobility of life forms and the ability to hunt for food. This created a challenge for life. If there was no mechanism to run from predators, eventually all of the creatures will perish because the predators will feast on the prey and eventually they would run out of prey since all the prey were so easy to hunt. When they did, predators would have nothing to eat. So, to balance out the predator and prey dynamics, fear came into the collective neurology. With fear, animals were motivated to run or fight (commonly known as fight or flight). Fear is such a primary emotion that it sits at the base of the brain. All other neurological additions evolved after that and sat on top of it. The fear center sits at the base of the brain and it grips all actions of the body and acts as a filter for all other thoughts and decisions.

With respect to hunger, fear plays a critical role. All else being equal, without food, the body perishes. And if it misses a meal or two it starts to wonder if food is coming at all. It creates a fear in the system and the one way to alleviate that is to fulfill the desire for food. Hunger releases a burst of energy that allows the person to go out and look for food - same in animals.

This is why, to be successful, they say you have to be hungry, that way you get the energy to move and act. When that desire is fulfilled, the fear is suppressed and the primitive brain rewards the conscious part of the brain with dopamine neurotransmitters. This results in a feel good moment and slowly that develops into a habit.

Fasting changes all these mechanisms and returns the body to the proper state. When you fast, the initial reaction is overwhelming. The primitive part of the brain raises all kinds of issues. It causes you to imagine death, or permanent health issues, or fainting. The number of fears that crop up for the beginner is as varied as you can imagine, but none of these are real. It is just the primitive psyche throwing a fit. When you fast, the first thing you benefit from is knowing your own limits and you start to know which voice within you to believe. You soon learn, when you fast, that you are much stronger and more resilient than you thought before.

Your body is not a fixed system, it works by replacing things over time. Even the hardest part of your teeth is subject to renewal and so are your bones. You shed skin on a daily basis and that is regenerated from the inside. All these systems and tissue need to be replenished, just like your enzymes, and even your blood cells and immune system. That replenishment comes in the form of nutrients. That's why you can't just live on sugar alone, because you may get all your energy from the sugar, but in time, you will not be able to replace the parts of you that were utilized and you will start to lose functionality in those systems and start getting ill. You need a balanced intake of energy and nutrients. If you had to pick what to focus on, choose the nutrients because nutrients have calories, while calories alone (like that from corn syrup) can be empty calories.

When you take the pleasure of eating out of the equation, there is an ingenious system at work that most of us do not know about. We indulge in all kinds of fad diets and we end up paying the price in terms of health and side effects, but all we have to do is let the body do its thing and you will be healthy.

The body has a finely tuned system of intake and energy creation. The body has three sources of energy to choose from.

The first is the food that has just been consumed. In this metabolic pathway, the body goes after the nutrients that were most recently consumed. It absorbs the nutrition and that nutrition is taken directly up by the blood stream and sent to all the systems that require energy. The brain is the first system that gets the intake because, in all your body, the brain is the system that has the highest consumption of energy.

From there it goes to all your other vital systems. But in the event that the body is not able to take on food, it goes to fat stores. Fat is just energy that is stored in the dermal layers and in other places. The metabolic pathway to consume this fat is different from the path to consume the energy in the food that is consumed. The body that is untrained takes a long time before it can switch from one source to another. Most athletes have trained their bodies to go from one source to the next in fairly rapid processes, but still, it is an uncomfortable one and one that serves a purpose.

When long distance runners complete utilization of the food they most recently consumed, they need to switch pathways and the point when they switch is what they call hitting the wall. It feels like a total depletion of energy and the onset of passing out. It suddenly feels like they have no energy whatsoever. They could even feel like vomiting and even passing out. Then they get their second wind and there is a sudden feeling of wellness and an energized state. It is easier to reach this energized state when you are up and about and in a state that tells the body that you are in need of the extra energy. If you spend your time resting and sleeping, the switch to the fat burning metabolic pathway is not forthcoming.

It takes a long time to complete the fat burn. The body goes through the entire system, systematically targeting areas that hold on to fat and converts it for utilization. You will feel a sort of mental clarity when you start burning fat. The brain seems to power well when you convert fat for energy and it develops a sense of focus that is unparalleled.

The third source of energy, and this can be targeted even while the fat is being burned, is the muscles. Muscles are targeted on a frequent basis to feed the body with amino acids required by essential systems. This is the reason you work out the breathing muscles and the ambulatory muscles so that they are not targeted for conversion. When you work them out they don't atrophy and that way you do not lose muscle mass from those areas.

So, there are three sources of energy that the body will go after. The first is the store in the stomach, the food you ate during your last meal. The second is the fat stored in your body, and the third is the muscle mass that you have, especially the muscles that are not of primary importance and the ones that you are not using.

Water

During the fast, and beyond, you do need to drink lots of water. This is a serious matter and dehydration should never be a part of your fasting. You need to drink more water when you fast because the body will be flushing a lot of waste out of your system. When fat is burned, there is a large amount of waste material that is generated and needs to be filtered by the kidneys. In the event there is insufficient hydration, the kidney could start having problems.

Don't wait till you feel thirsty. Once you feel thirsty, it's too late. The body is reliant on water and is more sensitive to its scarcity. You can live between 35 to 50 days without food, but you won't get past Day 6 without water.

When you are on a fast you need to pay attention to your water. Avoid RO water and regular tap water. Your best bet is a reputable bottler of mineral water. When you fast, it is important to be hydrated and sustain the mineral that you have in your body. RO Water is almost pure, meaning there are no dissolved minerals in it, and because of water without any minerals in it acts as a sponge, they leech minerals from the body when they enter our system, and take it with them when they exit the system

When we fast, the idea is to reprogram the body and mind to manage its resources on its own but not to remove resources from it. RO water, for instance, removes almost 99% of the calcium and magnesium that regular water would contain. So when it enters the body, this 'empty' water will leach calcium and magnesium from your system among other minerals. So stay away from RO water when you are fasting.

Mineral water, on the other hand, that is not fortified or processed in any other way except for the removal of pathogens, bacteria, and heavy sediments is what you should be looking for. If you have a filtration system at home or you are confident of the filtration process of your municipality, information of which you should be able to find online, you can boil the water and set it aside to cool before consumption.

Convenience

We've seen what the mind, body, and spirit are like and how we have evolved to a point where food is now by the clock and not when necessary. It would be rather strange to think that our ancestors who lived in caves decided to go out and hunt for lunch the moment they saw the sun hanging on the zenith. It didn't work that way.

Our bodies acclimatized to scheduled meals. Meals became part of our itinerary and so our habits evolved with that. Those eating habits were convenient, especially to make room for organized labor schedules, but they really didn't mean anything for our health or for our sustenance.

If you look at any diet that is grounded in fact, you will understand that the whole point is trying to maneuver the intake, but they still continue to frame it within the context of a three-meal day. We look at the opportunity to cut out fats, we look at the opportunity to cut out carbohydrates and we even talk about cutting out sweets. But the problem is that all these are based on the state of food as we know it.

Food is no longer the natural source of energy that we once evolved with. Food has become processed for taste and convenience, preserved for packaging, and colored for appeal. Food is no longer food; it is a package of marketing principles. Our body adapts to it and then we find that the long term effects include illness on one hand and habitual eating on the other. We get into this cycle of unhealthy consequences.

For most people, the fasting process is more mentally abrasive than physically restrictive. By embracing fasting, they suddenly remove the shackles of their indoctrination and start to see the value of themselves.

Aerobic Vs. Anaerobic Exercise

When you fast, it is important, in fact, it's imperative, that you work out consistently and intelligently. Why? Because fasting is not just about losing weight or learning to take control, it's also about reprogramming habits of the mind and processes of the body. When you work out, that becomes a habit too, and when you work out in the fasting state, the body's use of energy should be done in a way that inflicts less strain on the body, which means you should rely on aerobic exercise.

The benefit of exercise when fasting is magnified and you should take advantage of it. But more importantly, your body is genetically designed to be active even in the midst of zero food intake. Just be cognizant of the quality of your workout. To do that, you have to understand the difference between aerobic and anaerobic metabolisms and how you can use it to your benefit.

The preference is to use aerobic means of respiration in all states, fasting or otherwise. But sometimes the aerobic means takes time, and many times we don't have all the time to get a boost of energy. So our body has the mechanism of anaerobic respiration where there is no need for oxygen. But this only comes in short bursts, like running the 100-meter sprint from a dead stop. The body has this back door to energy reserves in case of emergencies, but those sources of energy are for quick and short instances. When you are fasting, you don't want to tap these sources.

However, there are also times when the increased breathing is insufficient to deliver the oxygen that is needed to the cells in the muscles. In this case, the body switches its dependence on anaerobic respiration and this should be avoided as well, if possible. As such, when you work out during your fasting days, work on matching your breathing to your workout intensity. This way you can extend your

workout and build your stamina and keep a consistent
burn rate.

**

Chapter 4 Preparing for the Fast

There is a huge cloud of mystery of what fasting is and what it does for the human body, the evolving mind and the divine soul. The only way you can draw back the curtains and see what fasting actually does is if you do it yourself. This book is written with the intention that we bring you as close to the water as possible, whether you drink, is up to you.

A Holistic Look at Fasting

Fasting is, in a way, about paying it forward. You have to undergo the pain and desperation and go against all the senses of your body telling you that you're wrong. It's the same voice that tells you that you were designed to eat three squares a day and that fasting is unnatural. The moment you hear that voice, you know that you are being led down the primrose path. It's easier to go with the flow and abandon all notions of fasting, but I want to tell you that you need to stick to it. You need to go through with it. The only reason that fasting is not for you is if you are medically unfit to undertake this journey, and a competent doctor tells you so.

So, check with your doctor. Ask him if everything in here will work for you, then get started. But before you dive in, you need to prepare mentally and physically. It's like the thing athletes do before the game. You got to get psyched, get stoked, and get pumped.

Preparation

Once your doctor gives you the green light, it's time to jump in, but jump in with preparation. You need to prepare for the journey. If you don't do the necessary preparation, the experience could be unpleasant and perhaps put you off of fasting for some time to come, not to mention the fact that you could have some unhealthy consequences arising from sudden fasting.

If you have a target date for fasting, then you need to back up from that date by two weeks and start your prep. Preparing for a fast just means that you get your body hydrated and you cut down on the processed foods.

If you are wondering what processed foods have to do with the price of tea here, well the thing is that processed foods are addictive in the most insidious way. You may not realize it, but the reason you keep going back for more and you keep loading your grocery cart is because you are already hooked.

Processed foods contain ingredients that are designed to appeal to the senses, but not necessarily provide you with the nutrients that you need. You read earlier in the book about the balance between nutrition and calories. Processed foods are low in nutrition but high in calories, and they are addictive to boot.

So in the lead up to the fasting exercise, switch your body from anything that makes it dependent, and look to hydrate your body. If you are dependent on something, then when you fast, it gets that much harder to go without the food. So when you hit the craving, you're going to think that's hunger and it gets harder to keep fasting.

But if you phased out the processed food, your body gets a chance to wean itself off the addictive foods and so when you get to the fasting stage, you only need to contend with laying off food in general.

Chapter Four Take Away

If you are fasting for the first time, it's going to be challenging because the mind is not going to be comfortable with it. The ability to fast is controlled by the mind, specifically the primal instincts of the brain. To change your life in other areas you need to learn how to control this part of you. When you fast, you find the answers and the methods to bring this part of you under control.

Chapter 5 The Fast

Before we get started, let's remember that the purpose of fasting is to:

1. Return your body to the powerhouse that it is without the excess intake of food. Let us remind ourselves that by fasting you are empowering and fine tuning the systems of your body.
2. Realign your mind and discipline its misconceptions accumulated over the years.

Let us remember that fasting cleanses our bodies and brightens our mind. That mind is one of the most important aspects of our evolution because it provides the bridge between the spirit inside us and the world outside. It is the mind that can take the inspiration of the soul and convert that intangible into the work of art for all to experience. The mind is what we are all about and fasting does more for the mind than it does for the body.

The goal is to make small incremental changes from one day to the next. The goal is to keep up the march and make it a marathon and not run it as a sprint. Fasting is a long haul endeavor and will return results in ways that you can't imagine in the short term and ways you have not even begun to fathom for the long haul.

If you have jumped ahead to this and skipped the pre-fast program, I strongly urge you to go back and condition your body to get to this stage. If you don't, you will be faced with other withdrawal symptoms and that could make the first three days very hard and even possibly be a stumbling block for most of you.

Day One

This is the first of three days that will result in the most changes to your body. It is going to be the hardest fight you've ever encountered, but as the Romans used to say, "*vincit qui se vincit*", which loosely translates to, "*he who conquers, conquers himself*". This is the battle of all battles that you need to wage, and win, to be able to step into the light of knowledge that you are the master of all things – that happens when you are able to conquer yourself. It starts with you beating the greatest habit of all - the strength to beat back the desire to eat.

I find it best to start the fast by skipping your dinner on T -1 (the day before you start the full day of fasting) and going to bed. That way, the first stage is a little gentler on your psyche since you will be asleep most of the night and you will wake up fresh to a body that has already entered the fasting state.

On Day One, you've already used up all the energy from your last meal. As you slept, the last sources of glycogen stored in your liver from that meal had also been used up. Now your body needs to find a new energy source. You are in a new state from the time you woke up on T0 – a fasting state.

In this fasting state, the body is going to do one thing, and the mind is going to do something completely different, but both go about their own way of fixing the same problem. If you can detach your mind from the apparent discomfort, you will learn how your mind works under stress.

What you have to learn about your mind and body is priceless, and that is one of the benefits of fasting.

Day One Observations

The fasting state is going to do three things, and you just have to sit back and observe.

1.   The body is going to go down a cascade that it is genetically programmed to do to get to its next available source of energy. It will first go for the low hanging fruit, which is the food you just consumed.

Then it goes for the glycogen in your liver. When both of those are depleted in about 12 hours from your last meal, maybe 16 – 18 hours if you were sedentary or asleep, then your body goes into a new state called the fasting state. The fasting state is characterized by the body's source of food which is no longer external to the body. The source of food is now internal. There are two sources that it will attack – adipose tissue and muscle mass.

2.   Next, the mind is going to come online because it is going to interpret the cessation of ingested food as an unfulfilled habit. As much as we like to blame the body for causing the problem, it is not accurate to blame the body. It is actually a part of the brain located at the base called the amygdala that is starting to activate other areas of your brain and communicates to the system that a habit is not fulfilled. The human body's habit mechanism uses the carrot and stick approach to everything.

Once you have a habit, at the end of fulfilling it, you get a neurotransmitter bonus – you feel good. That good feeling then strengthens the habit. That's the carrot. If the habit is not fulfilled, the base of the brain creates an increasingly uncomfortable sensation. It results in a visceral sensation and a mental sensation of the feeling of despair and fear. What you have to do is understand that the brain is doing exactly what it has to, and in time, it will learn that this fasting is better and its own interest.

3. Finally, you will observe that reasons and rationalizations of the higher mind come into play. You will start to question, you will start to doubt, and you will even start to feel that death is imminent. None of this is true of course, and if you are not sure, go visit a doctor and do a work up to assure yourself it's not as dire as it feels. But the one thing you cannot do is give in to the chatter and the discomfort. Because that's all it is.

The key to fasting is to keep the distractions to a minimum. Change your routine and make your mind focus on something else. The first time I embarked on an extended fast, I didn't have any expectation of what my mind was going to do and was unprepared.

The second time I preempted the discomfort by keeping myself occupied on a project. That made all the difference.

The third time I did an even longer extended fast, I traveled to Bali. I had never been there before and so everything from the sights, to the sounds, to even the smells were different and I could tell that my mind was so preoccupied with everything that it did not even consider the discomfort of not fulfilling the habit of eating.

If you are wondering if you are going to have to travel every time you do a fast, don't worry you don't have to. I did it as an experiment and as a way to find distractions for my mind. Once you prove to your brain that fasting is ok and that there are rewards to it, the brain catches on pretty quickly and slowly puts you in a state that is more amenable to cycles of consumption/fasting.

When you wake up on Day One, you are going to be in a fasting state. If you are not, you will be soon enough. Different people take varying times to go from a digesting state to a fasting state. But that variance has its limits, it doesn't go much more than 12 hours from your last meal. By the time you wake up on Day One you've been without food for almost 18 hours.

Start the day with a glass of water. Two glasses, if you can handle it. Give your body enough liquids to keep the kidneys flushed. When you start to burn fat in a state of ketosis, your kidneys will end up working overtime if you are not drinking sufficient water. If you keep well hydrated before entering the state of ketosis, then the kidneys will be unaffected, but mind your water. Remember to heed the advice about water back at the end of Chapter 3.

There is nothing else for you to do but get on with your day and you want to set off on an advantageous footing. The last thing you want to do at this point is to remain sedentary.

Day One Work Out

You need to be able to work out and get your body consuming energy before it slows down the energy conversion temporarily. That will happen sometime on Day 2 for most of you. If you have an extremely slow metabolism, it might even happen as late as Day 3.

For now, start your body on exercises that are aerobic in nature.

In my personal experience, I found that a walk in the morning when the air is fresh, followed by a build up to a run or if you would rather cycle, do that instead. But whatever it is, start with some aerobic exercise before going into a heavier workout and ending with strength training. When you do strength training, you should focus on your leg muscles, your upper body muscles, including your arms, and your diaphragm.

Stop to drink water as many times as you can.

Your aim in keeping a workout regimen throughout the fasting period is to expand your body's capabilities that have been suppressed for some time. Genetically you are built to be able to extract energy for strenuous activity, but since you haven't done that in some time, you need to get back to getting used to it. The way to do that is by working out. The second goal of hitting the gym on Day One is to get you to expedite the onset of ketosis. This happens once glycogen in the liver and other organs are exhausted.

Ketosis is the stage when the cells start to use fatty acids to fuel activity instead of glucose. But this process takes some time to get up to capacity. In many people, it takes about a day for ketosis to generate enough energy to supply your cells with the fuel it needs for normal human activity. To cover the temporary deficit, the body turns to amino acids and a process called catabolizing. In this process, the body takes the amino acid in muscle tissue and sends it to the liver for a process called gluconeogenesis – a process to make glucose. This is when there is a reduction in muscle mass, but the reduction is minimal – a total of approximately 90 grams of protein is used, which works out to be about 3 ounces of muscle tissue.

By the middle of the day, you will have significant urges to eat. You should look at these urges closely because they are not originating from your stomach, although you feel the pangs in the abdomen area. You hear the sounds and you feel the remorse of getting on this diet. All your emotional responses are totally understandable. This is how your body is built because you have one trait – habits.

Habits force you to do things that you regularly do, and the body, or the conditioning of the brain, is that these things you do regularly are good for you. But with study and experiments, we know that eating three square meals a day is not the healthiest thing in the world.

Day Two

By the time you wake up on Day Two you will probably find yourself feeling less energetic but still in fairly good spirits. No food has passed your mouth in about 36 hours and you have been fasting for at least 12 hours at this point. This is the most important day in your fasting schedule. This is the day you will feel weak and this is the day that most people give in to their cravings. This is the day you need to be the strongest.

Start your morning with two glasses of water. You need to get as much water in today as possible in anticipation of your ketosis. You also need it because today you will start to feel dry in the mouth. So keep hydrated and that will also help to keep your tummy physically full. Whatever you do, do not cheat today and do not sneak in any food or beverage. Not even coffee and not even lemon in your water. You are at the cusp of ketosis and showing your body (for the first time) that you can force yourself over this wall.

All you need to think about is this - "ONE MORE DAY"- always postpone any desire to quit and remember that in the grand scheme of things one more day always passes very quickly. The changes in your perception of time notwithstanding, you will get to the finish line, and, at the very least, you just need to make it to the third day

What you need to do today is continue your workout. Do at least 20 minutes of aerobic workout and continue with some weights. You should also do a second workout in the evening. Stay hydrated and stay cool. Do not stay too long in the sun or in warm, stuffy places. If you are uncomfortable to be alone, you should have a friend be with you. This is more for peace of mind than it is for possible emergency.

If you feel sensations of nausea or light headedness, fret not. These are all normal issues that come with extended fasts. Your body is just trying to get your attention, or it is not used to it and it is going through withdrawal. What you need to do is let it pass. Like I wrote earlier, have someone with you for the first time and have them keep tabs on you. Once you get through the first time, and you're an old hat at this, you will sail through these days with no issues whatsoever.

If you are diabetic or if you are on any kind of medication, you should check with your doctor if things get out of sorts. Whenever I feel hunger or cravings I initially go for a full glass of water. I found out that cold water is not the best solution, and room temperature water did well for me.

Day Three

When you make it this far, you're probably going to make it to Day Six without too much trouble. Two things happen around this time. The first is ketosis. If you are not sure and would like to conclusively know, get to the pharmacy and buy a bottle of ketostix. Folks who are familiar with the Atkins Diet are probably familiar with this. The ketostix are little strips that detect concentrations of ketones in your urine. Just place them in your urine stream when you wake up in the morning. The build-up of urine in the morning after an overnight of accumulation is a better indicator of things. There is a color chart that's on the bottle, you can measure how dark the stick turns and cross reference that to how much ketones you're burning.

Now that you're in ketosis, your energy levels should be back up and you will begin to feel a lot less overwhelmed than Day 2, if it's not, just give it till tomorrow. Most people catch up by the third day or the fourth day at most. At this point, you should feel a sense of clarity – unless you're going through other forms of withdrawal. This is the reason it's important to go through the pre-diet plan. If you are having caffeine withdrawal or sugar withdrawal then that complicates the exercise.

The only way to move forward if you got these extra distractions is to be able to discipline yourself into not giving into food or beverage. Just remember, it's not the fast that's making it difficult, it's the other stuff. I know many coffee drinkers sneak in a cup just to get the caffeine, but you can't do that because it interferes with the shifting of metabolic pathways. You're either in or your out, don't straddle the half way line.

Besides your lack of lethargy and the entry into ketosis, your body is mounting an assault on the fat deposits around your organs. Research has found that there is significant reduction in deposits around the pancreas and liver and in key muscle groups around the third and fourth day.

Another thing that is stabilizing within you is the level of blood sugar and, even better, insulin levels as well. Stable insulin levels go a long way in promoting cardiac health and other serious health issues. You should also be feeling really great by the end of today (unless you have other cravings as mentioned.)

If you are worried about muscle mass loss, don't be. In people who do 30-day water fasts, research has shown they only end up losing a maximum of 2 – 2.5

pounds of muscle mass. At three days, you're doing fine.

The first time I was at Day Three I remember how confident I was feeling and how amazed I was at the level of alertness and the amount of confidence that just took me over. No one at work could tell that I was fasting, and neither could my trainer at the gym. I was feeling like I could do anything. From today till about the sixth day you will have temporary moments of cravings and doubt, but for the most part, you will start to experience total confidence.

End of the First Experience

If this is your first time experiencing fasting, it may be a good time for you to stop here. You would end on a high note and you will be able to return to regular food consumption by tomorrow after you start with small amounts of food. I will walk you through the breaking fast process in the next chapter. You are welcome, of course, to continue reading what it feels like going into Day Four through Six and how it feels from there on.

There are two things that you need to know in order to make an informed decision on if you should quit or keep going. The first is that if you are feeling generally good about yourself, but you only intended to do it for three days, there is nothing stopping you from going forward and take it all the way to seven days.

On the other hand, if you are struggling on the third day, then you probably have one of the body types that need to take it slow and build up towards a seven-day, or more, fast. Check back on your metabolic profiles in Chapter 1 and reassess your decision to keep going. Either way, if you've come this far, you have accomplished a major feat in your life and you deserve kudos and you should not put yourself down for not being able to continue or thinking about quitting.

If you do end today, it is absolutely fine. Your next step would be to come back and do it again in a month or so. Many people I know took years to build up to seven days. Some even took months to build up to three days. Baby steps. What counts is that you get there.

But whatever it is, you should continue reading so that you know what to expect and what to do the next time. If you were one of those people that have to stop at three days because other issues complicated the fast, like the need to have caffeine or you have a problem laying off the sugar, then you need to work on that.

There are two ways you can do that. One is that you go cold turkey. The other, gentler way is that you deal with those food addictions first. Get off the sugar and the caffeine first then come back and do the fast. Trust me, I know how it feels. I used to drink three cups of coffee by lunch and needed an espresso after lunch and another coffee by quitting time. My first fast was torture because I was caught in the need to have coffee. But I stuck to it with the stubbornness that I didn't want anything or anyone to control me. My parents could relate. I would not allow coffee to control what I had set to do.

My body fell in line and today I drink coffee when I want to, and when I don't, it doesn't bother me. I am no longer a slave to something that needs to be carried in a cup.

Day Four – Day Six

The three days from the fourth to the sixth day will be a breeze for most of you. By the time I got to my third fast, this fourth to the sixth day was invigorating. Your body has stopped thinking about hunger and it has moved on to a number of other things that will amaze you. I've even met a guy who swears that his eyesight improved after his sixth day the first time he did a seven-day fast. There are numerous stories of health benefits that were verifiable and even amazing to many people. But I can't speak to any of those. Even health gains that I saw in people I know personally are not something I can repeat because it's not a first-hand account and thus, open to question. I can, however, tell you some of the things that happened to me on the different fasts I completed – the 3-day, 7-day, and 23-day fasts.

It took me three years of fasting weekly before I mustered up the courage to commit for long fasts. In retrospect, it was never the physical issues, it was more mental than anything else. I wanted to do more than 21 but less than 30 for one specific reason, I wanted to see what benefits I could gain in a less-than-30-day stint.

If you have mounted the hurdle of any food or beverage addiction then what you are going to feel is the sheer exhilaration of a new body and a new mindset. The one thing that was almost hilarious was that I would start having thoughts of food. I was not hungry in any way. Stomach rumblings had gone on day three and whatever vestiges of light-headedness and lethargy were gone as well. But I would have thoughts of food. They were as plain as day and obvious that they were purely in my head. That's what was enlightening. My mind was trying to psych me into eating. I would think about the restaurants I'd frequent or the dishes I'd like to cook, even the kind of fixings we used to have at Christmas Dinner. That was my ghost, as I started calling it. These left on Day Six typically and were replaced by negative thoughts.

The other thing that happened in this period was that my tongue started to have a white coat that stayed until the ninth day for me. It happened every time. My doctor believes that it's one of the signs of toxin elimination. No matter how much I scraped my tongue and washed it, it remained. Be prepared for this and don't freak out. You will also start to have morning breath around the fourth day, but that goes away pretty soon. This is also a consequence of toxin expulsion by the body. For me, it's usually gone by the time the white stuff disappears.

The first time I did a seven-day fast, one of the things that didn't appeal to me was that bowel movement and evacuation ground to a halt. I was advised sometime later that using the aid of enemas during the first three to four days would have a great effect.

I tried that the next time when I did a 14-day fast. The effects were absolutely amazing. By the fifth day, after three days of enema, my skin looked and felt different. I lost an inch off my waist and my ability to focus skyrocketed.

One of the things that I fell in love with when fasting was that my ability to think and work just rose to a new level. Each new level was one that I had no idea even existed. Clearing the toxins from my stomach also had another effect that I was not expecting. After I completed the fast and went back to a regular one- (or two-) meal per day diet I was amazed to note that I didn't need large portions to feel satiated. You will feel this as well.

The reason this happens is that the body is now able to absorb nutrients at a better rate with a cleaner body. When you absorb nutrients well, you don't need more food to get to that point and that means you don't take in all those extra calories.

Working out was easy even up to the sixth day. If you can make it to this point, the rest will be easy if you can control your mind. From here on out, it's more psychology than physiology.

Day Seven

This isn't an exact science and each of us has different experiences, different genetics, and different perspectives. So when I say something happens on a particular day, it may happen a little sooner or a little later for you.

The seventh day was a bit of problem for me, and the first time I was doing this fast past the seventh day, the choppy waters took me back a bit. I guess its nature's way of cutting me back a notch because I was starting to feel cocky, I guess.

The morning of the seventh day began with a burning sensation in my stomach. It was an acidic feel that I had learned about and I was deluded in thinking that I had escaped this experience. The other times that I had gone up to the seventh day, it didn't happen, but this time it did and I was disappointed. I am not sure if I was more disappointed that I was no longer the super human I was starting to think I was, or whether the pain was annoying. A little of both. The thing that I want to tell you at this point is that getting over this is fairly easy. All it is, is an accumulation of acid in the stomach and to get rid of it, which you must, is to drink a large mug of warm salt water. This should trigger your gag reflex, and you should let it. If you don't gag, have another mug. Vomiting the acid in your stomach relieves all the discomfort. When you're done, drink plain water.

The other thing that happens at this point is that your body has accelerated its fatty tissue conversion and you actually start to feel energized. Your ketosis is usually at a maximum at this stage and you are in a good place physically. Pain from the bouts of stomach acid, which will stop by the time you get to the 14th day, relieve and there is nothing else really in your way at this point expect your mind.

This is where I learned the most about myself from the seventh to the fourteenth day. I underwent a thorough schooling about who I really was.

With the additional clarity, I was able to see all the BS that I had accumulated. It is funny how having a clear mind tends to negate the propensity to avoid or tell yourself untruths. Shakespeare should have included that when he said, "To thine own self be true", "... and when you can't, do a seven day fast."

There must be some kind of a link between shedding physical toxin and mental toxin, but they appeared at the same time for me, and it was the same for a number of my friends who did 30-day fasts. For those of you focusing on the weight loss aspect of fasting, the seventh day onwards is where this really starts to show the difference. My urine ketone levels were turning the stick purple and I was peeling away the pounds faster than a plastic surgeon could (just about). By the time I got to the second night, I was 13 lbs. lighter (6 kg).

Day Eight – Day Fourteen

By the time I got to Day Ten, the voices in my head turned silent and the clarity I had experienced before Day Seven was back and in full force. The best way to manage doubt, negative thoughts and voices, are to let them be and never try to stop them or engage them. Don't even force them out of your head. These voices are not real and need to be ignored if they are to leave.

My ability to focus was never the same again. I could sit down and do something, and all time would stop around me. This was a great feeling because I found that my ability to get things done was accelerating and the outcomes were always accurate. Things that felt like guess work were not guess work but spot on all the time. The mental aspects of the fast were nothing short of phenomenal.

They say that golf is a mental game. They must be right since I shaved 9 strokes off my game.

I used this time to reflect on my life and where I was going. My heightened clarity gave me insight into what was what. It allowed me to make decisions that impacted my life and made me who I am to this day, almost three decades later. One of the things that it did to me was to remove the sorts of fear that were unnecessary. We all have fear when we have no insight into the consequences of our actions. Fasting gave me the insight I needed, and that released my fear. It also allowed me more compassion. My critical nature in the past was replaced with understanding.

Day Fourteen to Day Twenty Three

In my case, I only missed going to the gym for my daily half-hour workouts once in the entire 23–day period. That was on Day Seven. I hit the gym every day in the morning for the rest of the days and I found that my initial struggle wasn't anything I couldn't overcome, but it did require extra effort.

Here is what you can expect when you get past Day 14. When the body has started to go into maximum ketosis, it's also burning some protein, but in order to keep that to a minimum, the body also targets all non-essential tissue in the body.

Any extra growths that can happen in the organs, or non-body tissue and even microbes, including bacteria and pathogens, all get chewed up and used up for energy. Not only do the toxins get flushed, the other stuff that is not supposed to be in the body gets converted to energy, and the waste products flushed out. This is one of the many reasons you should continue with the enema at least once in three or four days.

At the end of 23 days, I lost a total of 36 pounds and went from a 44-inch waist to 35 inches. The most fat loss in my body happened around my abdomen. My next long fast will happen in November this year, at which time I plan to take it all the way to 30 days, but I don't expect I will lose much around my waist. The purpose of the next fast is to map the limits of my mind then push that further.

Chapter 6 Getting Back to Food

Fasting is important, but breaking fast, especially after 23 days, and even after seven or fourteen, in fact, even breaking fast after three days, is an important event. You have to pay attention to what you are doing and you have to know how to go about it or you could land up in the ER.

Fasting is easy, but breaking fast needs an understanding of what to do. Technically my fast lasted till the 23rd day, but I didn't pass one morsel of solid food until the 32nd day. On the 24th day, I drank orange juice. All this while I was drinking 2 – 3 liters of water daily, and now I just substituted 1 liter of that to orange juice. You can choose between orange or lemon juice. I personally prefer orange juice, but if you like lemon juice, that's good too. You can also have both if you can't pick which you like better, but the one thing you should not do is add sugar in it, it has to be freshly squeezed. I chose organic oranges and pressed them myself. The pressing part was a calculated move because I've always liked the smell of freshly squeezed oranges. I increased the juice intake on the 24th day but kept the water intake the same. I still needed water to flush out my system. I had mine at room temperature. Experts say that you can add honey, but I didn't do that.

On the 26th day, I added vegetable broth to my intake. It was just boiled vegetables pureed and squeezed to remove the fiber. I was not in a rush to consume solids yet and I was in tune with my body at the time so I knew exactly what I wanted. You will be the same. If you find that your body is telling you something different from what I experienced, don't be afraid of differing to your body. If you can make it past 21 days, you will be in tune with what your body needs and can handle.

I kept on this diet until the 29th day, and only on the 30th day did I start to introduce sold fruits. So, for the last two days of the breaking period, I had fruits and vegetable soup if and when I felt hungry, which was about once or twice a day.

There is one more thing that I found helpful in my path to solid foods. I started consuming yogurt. Yogurt contains lactobacilli, and that helps to repopulate your gut so that your impending food intake can be adequately and efficiently absorbed.

When I got back to regular food, three things had become clear:

1.   My appetite was precise – my body knew exactly what it needed and my mind knew exactly how to interpret that need.

2.   I would only get the urge to eat every other day, and when I ate I was turned off by large portions of food and was delighted with simple food in small portions.

3.   I had zero desire for caffeine or sugar and had no addictions to any group or class of food.

Maintaining Your Progress

The true nature of fasting is to return the balance of the body, mind, and spirit to a point that is most beneficial to each individual's development and the development of the species as a whole.

Once you've completed the fast, your view of life is much clearer and how you've been treating your body, how you've been neglecting your mind, and how you were not in touch with your soul, will come into focus.

***

Chapter 7 Healing the Body

One's purpose in fasting is to heal the body. I find that the best way to look at fasting. Let's put aesthetics aside. I have never been known to favor aesthetics over content, and so weight loss and fitting into nicer clothes were never my payoffs. Fasting, for me, has been about keeping my body healthy so that I can extract more from it and convert that into achievements and successes that would otherwise be impossible to consider. Better body health leads to a stronger mind. That's a fact.

While fasting is commonly associated with benefits that accrue to the body, and not so much to the mind or spirit, those who have fasted according to the plan proposed in this book unanimously agree. It seems to be commonly held that fasting's only benefit is to shed the pounds - fast! Yes, there are weight loss consequences to fasting, but it's not the only one and it's not the way you think.

The primary goal of fasting is to allow two of the three systems of your existence - body, and mind, to realign. As you have seen, our ancestors, who scientists show are the cause of our current set of genetic makeup, had a cycle of food consumption and food starvation. Their bodies and ours are built to optimize itself for those conditions. We haven't evolved out of that yet and that is one of the reasons that we tend to gain an enormous amount of weight over time when we just eat three squares a day and then snack in between and then do less work in the acquisition of that food.

When the energy doesn't get used up, there is nowhere for the fat to go, and too much fat accumulation in too many areas over a long period is detrimental to the system that was designed for a different rhythm of things.

Fasting is not about mimicking our Paleolithic brethren; it's about resetting the system so that we can go back to a diet that parallels theirs in a way that is more acceptable to this day and age.

The fasting that we need to look at will change the way you feel and the way you look, but more importantly, it will change the way you think and the way you are inspired to move forward and create a life for yourself that is beyond anything you can imagine without the proper inspiration. That inspiration will only manifest when you change the way you manage your energy.

Fasting has numerous effects, and not just on the body. The exact extent really does defer from one person to the next. In general, here are just ten common effects fasting has on your body:

1.   Improves insulin sensitivity
2.   Improves metabolism
3.   Improves the quality of hunger
4.   Improves quality of appetite
5.   Improves absorption of nutrients
6.   Improves the immune system
7.   Improves skin condition
8.   Improves cell regeneration
9.   Prevents premature aging
10.   Reduces weight

These are just the positive effects fasting has on the physical body. There are other effects that it has on the mind which are covered in Chapter 8. These ten effects are just the ones that you feel directly after just three days. There are more benefits that have been recorded for those who have taken it up to seven days, and even up to forty days. In that list of ten, two need some explanation.

Improving Insulin Sensitivity
What is Insulin Sensitivity?

Insulin is a hormone that is released by the pancreas. Without getting too technical about it, think of it as a key that opens a lock. The lock, in this case, is the lock on the 'gate' that stands between your bloodstream and the cells that need fuel to do a task - in this case, they need to absorb the glucose that is in the bloodstream.

When the insulin is in the bloodstream, it attaches itself to the cells and unlocks the cells to accept the sugar from the bloodstream. When you are adequately sensitive to insulin, only a small amount is needed to bring the high levels of sugar in the blood down and moving into the cells. If you are insulin insensitive, the blood sugar levels stay high in the bloodstream.

Insulin sensitivity is a primary concern for everyone, regardless of their weight. If your body goes through multiple cycles of heightened blood sugar and the release of insulin, in time, the insulin stops affecting how the cells absorb the sugar and you become insulin insensitive.

Another scenario that is equally as bad is when your pancreas is surrounded by fat and has trouble releasing sufficient insulin. In this scenario, there isn't enough insulin to help the cells absorb the glucose from the blood stream. This results in a prolonged period of high blood sugar levels (hyperglycemia) which can result in other complications.

Effect of Fasting on Insulin Sensitivity

After 12 hours of fasting, the body begins to attack the glycogen stored in the liver to use as energy. Once that is depleted, the body then goes to the fat deposits in other parts of the body, especially the deposits that accumulate around the organs, including the pancreas. This has an amazing effect. When it clears the fat stored around the pancreas, the pancreas starts to function better and is able to produce sufficient insulin to help mop up the excess sugar in the blood. This alone has amazing results for those with insulin irregularities.

Time and again, research has proven that fasting and depleting the fat stored in the body helps the body to function better and puts less strain systemically throughout the entire body. It has been proven time and again that improving insulin sensitivity has been a consistent effect of fasting.

If you can combine this with reducing, or totally wiping out, processed sugar consumption, then the insulin levels also return to a normal level and that lower insulin in the blood reduces risk of heart and other organ failures. On the one hand, we want insulin to move sugar from the blood to the cells where it is converted to energy, but at the same time, we do not want too much insulin coursing our veins as it is not healthy for the organs and tissue in our system. So the best way to move forward after the initial prep period and the major fast is to stay off the sugar and foods with a high glycemic index.

As we unfold the secrets of fasting during the course of this book, you will also begin to see the benefits and the changes across all three elements. But for now, let's focus on the body and see the effects fasting has.

Fasting is not the same as diets. So the first thing you need to come to terms with is that fasting is not designed to just reduce caloric intake, it is designed to change the metabolic pathways of your system.

A metabolic pathway is a series of steps or chemical reactions that the body needs to take to convert food into a form that can be absorbed by cells at a molecular level. When you dine on pasta, it's not pasta that goes into your cells to provide it with energy. That pasta is made up of all kinds of different molecules, especially carbohydrate molecules, that are then converted to energy along a specific sequence of events that we call a pathway. So, the metabolic pathway is a specific series of events that takes the morsels off food and converts them into energy. It doesn't happen in one big leap, it happens in a number of small steps.

Improved Metabolism
The term metabolism is widely used and most of the time it just means the amount of energy that the body

can develop through its chemical processes, but there is more to it than that. Metabolism covers three functions that happen within the cell.

1.   The conversion of food/stored fat to energy

2.   The conversion of food/stored fat to proteins

3.   The elimination of the byproducts of energy creation

The energy of the food consumed is converted and used at the cellular level.

There is a lot of confusion about the state of metabolism in the period of fasting. The reason for this confusion is that the metabolic rate depends on how long you are fasting. If you are fasting for more than 15 to 20 days, then your body is going to have a significant reduction in metabolism to conserve energy. But on the other hand, after just 24 hours of fasting, your body will increase its metabolism because of the lowered insulin levels in the bloodstream, increased growth hormones and, from an evolutionary perspective, it creates the energy for you to mobilize efforts to hunt for food. Pretty ingenious, I think.

The Hardest Part of Fasting

If you are doing this and you are already past the first week, you can relate to what I am about to say here. The hardest part of fasting is the mindset that we bring to the table. You are not the only one. Millions of people come to the dinner table with everything except nutrition on their mind. They come to the table for family reunion. They come for pleasure in the taste and decoration of the food. They come for the habit, yet don't realize it. They come to fulfill their obligation to eat, even when they are not hungry. This is unhealthy and has consequences. When you are done with the fast, try to return to a more sensible pattern of eating and exercise.

The single most important aspect of coming to the table is for you to be able to think that you are coming there for nutrition. To think about food as just a way to fuel and repair your body is one of the most uninteresting things you can think of, but that is exactly what you are doing. It's time to have a food revolution and stop thinking about food as a source of pleasure and think of food as a source of life. Eating is part of the circle of life and it is this eating that allows us to go into the world to be more than we currently even think about.

Improved Appetites

We touched briefly earlier about appetites and we talked about cravings, especially in women who are gestating. If you've been pregnant, the chances are that you suddenly had cravings for some of the weirdest things you can imagine. Those cravings are a mix of psychology and physiology.

When one is gestating, their body is literally knitting together a new life inside. That new life requires all new parts and it is designed to get the building blocks from the host - the mother. Sometimes the host does not have what is needed so it sends the sensation to the brain for interpretation. The brain then interprets that requirement as a craving and the body goes in search for the source of that nutrient.

But that's just one step. The second step is that the brain needs to be able to interpret what the body is in need of. To do that it refers to its memory of past foods and looks for the food that contains what it needs. When it knows where to find that ingredient, the brain then invokes the feeling like it wants to eat that particular food/dish.

This process of identifying what the body needs on different days gets totally messed up, especially when processed foods are brought into the mix and when the body is fed a high level of junk. The best place to start when coming up with good nutritional habits is when the child is in the womb and when the child is newly born. What the mother eats goes directly to the child and this is a good way to get the child on track with the best diet possible.

It's when we eat for pleasure and we eat processed foods that we are unable to actually look for the kind of food that contains the healthy doses of nutrition that we need. That is the reason we need to reacquaint the body with good sources of nutrition and without the high doses of sugar that we so often find in processed foods these days. Once your body is reintroduced to better sources of high-density nutrients you start to build a new library of nutrient information and the ones that your body can turn to when it needs a certain nutrient.

Mindful Eating – Post Fast

After the fast period, when it comes time for a meal we are usually in a rush or we are busy doing something else. It's a source of entertainment and a source of pleasure. None of this actually aids in the process of eating healthy.

When you practice reduced food intake after the fast, you should shift how you see your meal and start to practice mindful eating.

Mindful eating is about being one with your food and focusing on the eating process rather than just stuffing yourself while you are doing something else. When you eat just twice a day, once in the mid-morning and once in the mid-afternoon, you should spend no more than 20 - 30 minutes in the process of consuming your food. You should do it in silence and you should absorb the experience.

This is not so much about having fun with your food but it's a process of getting intimate with your nutrition. Mindful eating will change your life when you do it in concert with Intermittent Fasting. You will find that your body adapts to the changes in your habits and the changes to the lack of pleasure motives the act of nutrition consumption.

Have Fun

Having fun is not a bad thing. There are so many things you can do in life that will give you pleasure, but you shouldn't look at all these things for pleasure for pleasure's sake. Driving to work every day is a mindful experience while you pay attention to your vehicle and the other drivers on the road.

You pay attention to your driving and your route to the destination, but just because you love racing cars on the weekend doesn't mean you need to drive fast on the road as well. Eating is about eating, having fun is about entertainment. Sometimes eating can be about fun, but that is the exception, not the norm.

If you do it this way, you will take off the fat, get back to your ideal weight, and be able to stay healthy.

The power of intermittent fasting is that it shifts your focus and your habits away from something that is unnatural and unhealthy. It takes your body's dependence on repeated introduction to food and puts it where it belongs, on the dependence on stored resources. It also puts you in control over the kinds of food and increases your reliance on a healthy appetite. The power of intermittent fasting is that it is a liberalizing endeavor that allows you to take control over your life.

Junk Food

You also need to get junk food off your grocery list. The term is used in this book without any sense of exaggeration. Junk food really is junk. They are loaded with calories and mind-altering compounds that give you a feeling of euphoria, all the while decreasing your health and altering your preference away from things that are healthy to things that are addictive.

***

Chapter 8 Strengthening the Mind

Fasting is usually taken to be an act to reduce weight, and if you go a few steps further, it is understandable that it also gets you healthier. We covered all that. The body certainly benefits from the fasting, but trying to comprehend how cessation of food raises the mind can be a stretch for most people. I see that.

But the biggest benefit of fasting is not accrued to the body, it goes to the mind. To understand how, a review of the brain, the mind, and the psyche are required.

The Brain

The brain is a fascinating organ. It is built in a way that doesn't resemble any other organ in the body in terms of the cells that come together for its function. What's more is that there are a couple of dimensions to the brain that is all a blur. Not to worry, we will get to that.

The brain, the mind, and the psyche are three concepts that confuse most of us into thinking that the terms are interchangeable and one means the other. I assure you, all are different, all are interdependent to a certain extent, and all behave uniquely over the course of our existence.

The brain is physical. If you were to approach it surgically, you will find that you could pick it up and it had physical presence. It had color, texture, and mass. The brain was just the apex of the central nervous system, which spread throughout the body. This system evolved from a very basic and rudimentary purpose over millions of years, to become what it is today.

In essence, the entire mechanism - the brain, the mind and the psyche are all interconnected in that they are tasked with doing one thing - and that is to fulfill the purpose of our earthly existence.

Most of us, over most of our individual lives, fail to realize that there is a distinct separation between thought, word, and deed. Deeds are the tangible actions that our body performs. The word, on the other hand, is partially tangible and stands at the juxtaposition of being a figment of thought and the reality of action. Finally, there is thought, while being very real to us, it is, in fact, intangible.

The brain is part of the central nervous system and sits inside the cranial vault. Every part of the brain is tangible and has physical form. There are four kinds of cells that distinguish the brain, the neurons, and the other essential parts of the central nervous system.

The brain operates by using electrochemical signals and processes to accomplish its tasks of controlling the rest of the body's functions. There are two main functions the CNS has to perform.

First, it connects sensors to the brain. This connection allows the brain to get information from a host of sensors that the body houses - from temperature sensors to touch sensors, taste sensors, and smell. Even sight and sound information are part of the information that is sent back to the brain along the nervous system. Once the data is in the brain, the brain decides how to manipulate its surroundings to be able to accomplish what it needs to. Once this decision has been made, the signals are sent back to the peripheral tools in the body to convert thought to action.

For instance, a sensation of hunger sent to the brain could trigger a thought process that will direct the body to go in search of nourishment. In terms of hunger, there is more than just one trigger. In the case of hunger, there is the real call for nutrition which creates a sensation of hunger, and then there is the habit of calling for food at a certain time of the day. Both are the result of neural pathways that have been created over time based on the actions that we subject ourselves to and the external lessons we learn of when is a good time to eat. The decision process to get to the point of foraging for food can be arrived in one of two pathways in this instance. There may be more. The point is that the same outcome can be reached along different paths of the neurons.

The Brain's Structure

The brain is three pounds of gray and white matter with the consistency of blancmange, a kind of French custard. It is 75% water by weight and 60% fat by volume. It consumes about the same energy as a 20-watt light bulb and uses 20% of the entire oxygen intake and also 20% of the blood flow. To supply that amount of blood, there is approximately 100,000 miles (that's not a typo) of blood vessels involved in the supply and return to and from the brain. The brain is a resource hog, consuming more resources than any other organ in the body. The gray matter in the brain consists of neurons, and is about 40% of the brain, while the other 60% is white matter, consisting of dendrites and axons, responsible for the transmission of data. There are three functional areas of the brain, the cerebrum, cerebellum, and the brain stem.

The Cerebrum is the largest of the three areas and is divided further into lobes for organizational and observational ease. The four lobes are the frontal lobe, the parietal lobe, the temporal lobe and the occipital lobe.

The frontal lobe is responsible for a vast array of different human thought and action. It is a major part of motor function, memory, judgment, and impulse control. It is also responsible for social and sexual behavior.

The parietal lobe is where the sensory information like touch and pressure is processed. It is also the place where taste is processed.

The temporal lobe holds the areas of hearing, long term memory and the ability to recognize faces.

Finally, the occipital lobe is the area for sight.

These are just some of the important areas that have been listed. There are much more that would exceed the purpose of this book if we were to elaborate further. Needless to say, the lore that we only use less than ten percent of our brains is patently false.

To be more detailed, there are other areas of the brain that we can separate our study into it. There are specific areas of the brain that we know varying degrees of information, but for the most part, science has a long way to go in objectively mapping our brain and understanding how it behaves. Here are just some of the areas you need to know about.

Cerebral Cortex This part of the brain is instrumental in our ability to remember, pay attention and remain self-aware. It is located on top of the cerebrum and made up of folded gray matter.

Corpus Callosum The two hemispheres of the brain are connected by one bridge that allows data to flow between the two. This is the corpus callosum.

Ventricles In the center of the brain mass is a pocket of cerebrospinal fluid. The fluid is found here, in the brain, and in the spinal column. It is produced by the choroid plexus, also located in the ventricles.

Thalamus The thalamus is located alongside the ventricles in the center of the brain mass between the two hemispheres. It is responsible for pain management and sensory detection.

Hypothalamus Regulates the metabolic profile of the person and manages the autonomic functions of the nervous system and controls the activity of the pituitary indirectly controlling body temperature, thirst, and hunger.

The brain's functions that have thus far been mapped by western medicine are strictly based on physical representation of cause and effect. This means that when they were mapping the brain they would test one area and observe the effect of it and consequently map that function to that area. In each person, the exact location of the control varies and each person has to be mapped for where a certain function is located exactly. The approximate area is what is known. The exact area has to be individually mapped if surgery is contemplated or using an MRI conducted with appropriate stimulation.

The Cells of the Brain

There are two broad classifications of cells in the brain and spinal column. The spinal column, although not considered the brain proper, is an extension of the brain in many ways. It is there to help transfer the information to and from the body to the brain. The two types of cells are the glial cells and the neurons.

The neurons in the brain are made up of three distinct sections. At the head are the dendrites that connect to other cells. The dendrites are like tentacles that branch out from one cell body that contains one nucleus. From this same cell body extends an Axon. This Axon can vary in length. At the end of the axon, there are axon terminals. Axons carry nerve signals to and from the cell body.

The glial cells are very different from the nerve cells of the neurons. They have no active part in the formation of cognition. Their only job is to keep everything in place. Glial cells amount to about 90% of the cells in the brain.

The Mind

Everything you read above describes the physical elements of the brain. The mind, however, is altogether a different business. As much as we use both terms interchangeably, they do not mean the same thing in any way. The brain, as you saw, is a tangible organ that you can touch and feel. The mind, however, is intangible, and is more of a mental construct, than a physical object.

The mind uses memory and extrapolation (which can be referred to as imagination) to develop a kind of pseudo reality within our head. The mind uses algorithms that are based on occurrences in the real world and then extrapolated to understand and predict an outcome.

What we retain in our brain and the method in which we retain it are not exactly how we think it is. For instance, what we see is not what we remember; rather, what we remember is an impression of what we see. That's how it is for most people. For the rare few who remember things as they see it, they are referred to as ones who possess photographic memory.

The same goes for what we smell, and what we hear. It is all subject to interpretation before it is stored. This is true no matter how vehemently you believe that you remember things the exact way they occur.

However, photographic memory can be learned and can be practiced. The real trick is not to possess photographic memory, which is on one side of the arc, or to have processed memory, which is on the other side of the arc. The trick is to have a healthy balance of both. This doesn't mean that sometimes you chose to remember some things one way and other things in another way. What it is, in reality, is that you remember all things in raw and processed form, but took what you saw to different degrees in two different phases of your brain.

The Taming of the Undisciplined Mind

Once you have your fast sorted out and you are getting comfortable with it, you need to begin the process of cleansing your mind. This should come in during the pre-fast to take the most advantage of the interconnected nature of the systems. But more importantly, during the pre-fast, you would be encountering withdrawal issues and that is the area of the mind. Mindfulness, and perhaps meditation, will go a long way in alleviating many of the adverse effects. We do this with mindfulness achieved through breathing exercises.

Stage 1 Breathing Exercise

The first stage exercise is meant to initiate you into a sequence of breathing and mindfulness exercises. There are four stages that you will go through before you begin to see the effects that will astonish you.

The beginning of Stage 1 is simple. Find a spot that you are comfortable with. Close your eyes. You have no other tasks to accomplish. All you have to do is watch your body breathe. When you do this with your eyes closed, it will seem as though you are watching from a point that is between your two eyes, just above the bridge of your nose in the middle of your forehead. It will only seem like this. Identify this as the seat of your Self.   Once you close your eyes and start watching your breathing, remember that that's all you need to do.

Remember to place all other distractions on hold. When you sit down and watch your breathing, count how long it takes to inhale. 1 Mississippi ... 2 Mississippi... 3 Mississippi... until your breath reaches the end of its natural cycle, and prepares to exhale. Remember, you are only watching, not controlling.

So whatever rhythm of breathing that is currently a part of you is what you are watching. Do not try to change it to inhale deeply or exhale fully.   When you do this, you will note the number of seconds it takes to inhale. Then count the time it takes to exhale. The time it takes to exhale, may or may not be the same time as the inhale, and for now, that does not matter. What you need to do is just be aware of the count. Keep doing this and focus on the breath and the count.   When you are done, open your eyes and relax in your same position and slowly let the rest of life enter your conscious observation. Listen to each sound as they enter your consciousness. Then open your eyes and let the information flood you. As you become aware of your surroundings, keep in mind only what you must. Because you have just begun to realize that when you are flooded with information, your mind can only pay partial attention to any one thing.

When you repeat this every day for a week, you will do two things: you will slow down your rhythm and you will peel away whatever stress you are currently facing, even if you didn't know you had any. But this is just the first part of it. To understand nature, slowing down is a major part of success.

Stage 2 Controlled Breathing

The second part is when you begin to control your breathing to match the inhale and exhale times by matching the times you are intentionally controlling your breathing. But do not jump to this step right away. You must take it slow. The chances are that you are like the 99% of people around the world and your breathing techniques are wrong, to begin with. If you learned to breathe right from young, your diaphragm will be strong and you can control your tempo incredibly well. As you practice this breathing technique, what you will slowly realize, aside from the better breathing habits and the calming of you mind, you will also notice that your extremities begin to tingle. It just means that your pulse oxygen level is going up. You are sending more oxygen to the rest of your body and they are literally waking up.

With this simple exercise, and without too much effort, you have already begun to cleanse your body and oxidize much of the gaseous toxins that are present. By doing the weekly water fast, you have also started to cleanse your gut, and by doing that, you have started to improve the quality of your blood. With the increased blood quality and the increased breathing, oxygen is going to be flowing in abundance, and your cells will begin to rejuvenate themselves.

Stage 3 Visualize Your Distractions

The third stage of meditation is going to be able to help you completely quit the habit of eating and get you on the road to health. The third stage is also rather simple and all you need to do is extend the time you take away for the purpose of meditation.

The idea here is to visualize your distractions, and eating is certainly a distraction. When you get to this stage, what you are doing is to acknowledge your distractions, but not taking part in them. You will find that your thoughts have a mind of their own. Those thoughts are beyond yourself, and what you are doing is separating yourself from random fragments of thought. Don't worry - everybody has them.

When you are watching your breathing, you will realize that you are able to monitor everything that goes on about you. The same thing is now expanded when you start to look at not just what you are doing with your breath, but also what you are doing within your mind. The thoughts that you have will be more visible to your mind's eye and you will be able to watch them go by without interacting with them. The benefit of this third stage is that you are becoming the master of your mind which means that you will be able to be less stressed in many situations. To really reap the benefits, you should keep going and never stop the daily meditation routine and the weekly fasting. Just as fasting and veganism cleanse the body, mindfulness, and breathing exercises clean the mind.

The mindfulness exercises that you have been practicing allow you to remember one salient truth, that the past and the future do not matter and what does matter is the moment. Being mindful is about being in the moment. Being in the moment is the most important thing in the world when you are trying to do anything in this world.

Stage 4 Instantaneous Focus

When you get to this stage, the idea is to be able to control your breathing at the drop of a dime - to control what your mind is doing at the drop of a dime - to control where you are in a moment. Once you can do all that, you have reached the pinnacle of the simple meditation. There is no need to visualize anything. Your breath is the most powerful thing in the world. Between your mind, and your breath, there is almost nothing that you cannot cure.

In stage four, it is time to move your meditation to other parts of your life. Wherever you are, pay full attention to what you are doing. Wherever you are, make sure you are in the moment, especially when you are eating. Whether you are on the bus, on a plane, be mindful. Being mindful is not about being withdrawn. You are fully aware of all that is happening around you, you are just not participating, but you are watching.

Meditation has a multidimensional effect on everyone. It is one of the best ways to get in touch with what is going on inside you. With mindfulness exercises and breathing exercises, one of the benefits you will begin to experience is that your body will tell you what it needs. With this and the upcoming effects of fasting, you are going to experience a new dimension of control over your life.

This will result in you getting visions of what is necessary and what you need to eat. It will be the way your body tells you what it needs from a nutritional standpoint. When you combine fasting with meditation and mindfulness, what you end up doing is getting in touch with your body and understanding what your body wants.

Your mental health and framework is an important aspect of all things that you do. When you embark on a quest for a healthier life and a more finely tuned body, mindfulness in all that you do will only take you to higher accomplishments. Being able to counter the temptation cultivated from decades of incorrect eating patterns is better handled with the aid of meditation and mindfulness.

***

Chapter 9 Energizing the Spirit

Fasting sheds the toxins in the body, which in turn clears the mind. The will necessary to implement the fast strengthens the mind and diminishes the idle chatter that an undisciplined mind will naturally do. The mindfulness exercises help to channel the energies, and that results in a quieter and more focused mind.

All this serves to do nothing to the soul, except move out of its way. Changing your mindsets, altering your body's health and silencing the mind's unnecessary musings don't affect the soul. What they do is silence all the things that have been thus far obfuscating the soul's constant presence and attempts to communicate with you.

Your soul (for lack of a better description of the energies that are at the core of your being) is the same energy that makes up the fabric of the universe. When you hear about things like the Law of attraction and having the universe grant you all your desires, that is the universe that connects to your soul. It doesn't just connect to it, it is it.

When you fast, you open up a channel, cutting through the thick layer of junk that filled your body and mind. Fasting removes those things that prevented you from clearly communicating your desires and blocked you from the inspiration of the soul that answered your desires. If you haven't been able to get the Law of Attraction to work for you, this is the missing puzzle.

There is nothing you can do to change your soul. Fasting doesn't change it, fasting just clears up your mind and body so that you can hear the silence of the soul loud and clear. When you do, clarity becomes an everyday event for you and fear evaporates.

Conclusion

The key to life is indeed balanced. Not just in the intake of energy and the use of it, but also in the level of contribution each part of your existence has on the trajectory that you take in life. A balanced life has pleasure in life and the achievement of the mind together, under the inspiration of the soul. The only way to achieve all three states to work in harmony is through fasting.

Thinking about fasting in terms of aesthetics is fine to an extent, but it is a significant underestimation of all that fasting can do for you. You just have to be open to its power and its consequences.

In this sense, fasting is about balance. With the proper balance, you will be able to fulfill your dreams and purpose in life.

The initial fast that you do helps you to return to the balance you need to experience life beyond the simple cycles of eating and working to feed yourself.

Fasting is a comprehensive strategy to experience a better life. It takes time and patience and it takes will. You have one life to live, you should make the most of it, and fasting opens that door for you.

I wish you the best in your journey to fasting and clarity. May you find what you are in search of and let it be all you hoped it would be.

***

Congratulations! You have now learned how to heal your body, sharpen your mind, and reenergize your spirit through the miracle of fasting! If you enjoyed this book, a review would be much appreciated. Thanks in advance!

Intermittent Fasting Guide: Super-Charged Results for Energy, Health, and Weight Loss

Intermittent Fasting Guide: Super-Charged Results for Energy, Health, and Weight Loss

Includes 30 Recipes and an Intermittent Fasting Meal Plan

Kyle Faber

Intermittent Fasting Guide: Super-Charged Results for Energy, Health, and Weight Loss

Heal Your Body Through a Return to Healthy Eating Patterns

Copyright © 2018 Kyle Faber

All rights reserved. No portion of this book may be reproduced, stored in a retrieval system, or transmitted in any form or by any means – electronic, mechanical, photocopy, recording, scanning, or other – except for brief quotations in critical reviews or articles, without prior written permission of the publisher.

Published by CAC Publishing LLC.

ISBN 978-1-948489-97-3 paperback

ISBN 978-1-948489-96-6 eBook

This book is not intended for the purpose of providing medical advice.

All information, content, and material of this book is for informational purposes only and is not intended to serve as a substitute for the consultation, diagnosis, and/or medical treatment of a qualified physician or healthcare provider. The reader should always consult his or her healthcare provider to determine the appropriateness of the information for his or her own situation or if he or she has any questions regarding a medical condition or treatment plan.

Chapter 1: Why Intermittent Fasting?

The Human Inheritance

How we eat has a direct impact on how we think, how we feel, how long we live, and how we influence our progeny. The bulk of this book is intended to unravel why we eat the way we do, why we really should change that to eat in a way that helps us reach our full potential – and how intermittent fasting can help us do that.

Before we can really talk about intermittent fasting, we need to begin with two premises. First, our human physiology is the aggregate result of the environments around us. Those environments include the physical environment, the elements and nature; the psychological environment, our thoughts and feelings; and the intangible environment both within and surrounding us. Second, we are the culminative result of the generations that have come before. The human mind, body, and spirit are like an organic blockchain (to borrow a term from a technology). We have been impacted by and are the result of what our predecessors did as far back as the first single-celled organisms. Conversely, each thing we do now will have an impact on the generations to come.

So, let's start with a little history and look at how we evolved to get to where we are now.

Human beings weren't always the dominant species on the planet, and our ancestors were not always at the top of the food chain. Everything we now take for granted, from buildings that scrape the sky, to the planes that fly across it, to writing and computers and all the technological and scientific advances of mankind, are all things that have happened in the last 10,000 years. That may seem like a long time because our average individual lifespan is a mere 0.007% of that, but 10,000 years is a drop in the bucket compared to the 6 million years it has been since humans were arboreal, or the 20 million years that it took human beings to stand upright as we do now.

As human beings evolved, so did their eating habits. At some distant point in our common history, our ancestors began to change the way they consumed their nutritional requirements. Whether by necessity or opportunity, mankind shifted from being scavengers to becoming hunter-gatherers. They stopped needing to raid the carcasses of larger prey after the lions and hyenas had had their fill.

Then, as our ancestors developed tools and fire, their eating habits changed even more, and human beings were catapulted to the top of the food chain. Once they began cooking food, early man was able to eat less, because more was nutritionally available from each portion of food, and because cooked food needed less digestive processing, that energy was redirected to cognitive development.

It turns out that we owe much of our intelligence to man's mastery of fire and becoming able to cook our food! As our brains grew, we no longer needed to scavenge the food that other animals, like lions, hunted. We started making tools, and extended our abilities further using external objects. Not only did we diversify our sources of energy – fruits, seeds, berries, and whatever we could gather in the fields and forest – but we could now organize and hunt prey of our own. By the time the Paleolithic age rolled around, we had graduated to being hunter-gatherers, hunting prey and gathering food. As the quality of our food increased, mortality rates decreased, and human populations increased.

Hunting and gathering also played into a new pattern that was forming – our ancestors began to travel. They would harvest all they could from wherever they were, and when there was nothing left to forage, they would pack up and leave in search of the next area that would offer them bounty. A nomadic strain was added to our genes, becoming another part of our heritage. Small groups would forage a location, exhaust all it had to offer, and then move on to the next spot. Two key developments happened in this line of humans: first, their eating patterns became entrenched in human biology, and, second, they started forming organized groups.

The bulk of the nutrition consumed by our biological ancestors came from meat they hunted, supplemented by the seeds, fruits, grains, and roots they found in the areas they settled in. For a million years, the majority of their energy needs was supplied by prey – meat. What they ate, when they ate, and how much they ate helped shape human physiology of eating and digestion, and the distribution and use of energy and nutrients in the human body all the way into the modern era.

Most importantly, our ancestors experienced feast or famine as the overriding pattern of the day. With no refrigeration or no other technologies to stop the decay of meat after slaughter, these hunter-gatherers had two options. They could either eat everything or let it rot. So they would eat everything and share their food with the whole community. Whenever there was meat from prey, they feasted. That would be a high protein meal with a high fat content. When there was no prey to provide that meat, they had little to nothing to eat.

Over time, the human body of our ancestors adapted. Their metabolic processes adapted, developing an efficient way to handle cycles of feast and famine. The human body developed a more robust fuel tank system. Of all the food that they ate, which was large in quantity during times of abundance, some was converted to glycogen for liver and muscle storage, and the rest was converted into fat and distributed over the body. It is an efficient system. Instead of having a single storage location, the human body uses the surface layer under the skin, an expandable and contractible organ, to store the fat as it became available. The human body also kept some readily available energy in the form of glycogen in the liver and muscles. That could be easily converted to fuel when needed. The rest of the stored energy would need to go through a specific metabolic cycle to convert the stored fat back into usable energy.

On the day after a feast, the group wouldn't need to hunt, and they would be full and satiated. The body would divert its energy resources from the brain and the limbs to the digestive system to aid the process of digesting all that food and the distribution of those nutrients and fats. This would be a basically lazy day. If they needed something else to sustain them, they still had things like fruits and seeds to eat.

During those first hours, energy in the form of glycogen would supply their basic energy needs, from keeping their brain functional to having energy available for defense if needed. However, that glycogen source was not designed to last very long.

Once it was depleted, the body would switch to using the fat stored subcutaneously. At that point, the satiated and related feelings from the feast would dissipate as the byproducts of the alternate fat-burning metabolic processes would begin to fuel their brains – and that would be like a shot of caffeine.

All this meant that an early hunter-gatherer had two tools that allowed him to rapidly climb to the top of the food chain. First, he had a significant amount of energy to draw from – more than just the glycogen stores that fed him during the first day after the feast. He had pure concentrated energy in the form of fat that could be converted back into energy to power his muscles. A byproduct of that conversion, ketones, could power his brain, giving his brain an extra boost. The combined effect of increasing muscular power (resulting in speed and endurance) and a more robust brain allowed early man to outsmart his prey and have the energy to outrun his prey. While man was not faster than most of the prey he targeted, he was certainly smarter and could keep going even after the animal became incapacitated from exhaustion.

That is our human legacy. That is the way our bodies and brains have evolved. We have the potential to power our brains and our intelligence, and the power to have strong and resilient bodies – if we manage our energy profiles correctly to take advantage of that legacy.

But our human history didn't end there. Our ancestors continued to develop. They learned the benefits of living in larger groups, and started to learn how to farm. Farming allowed them to stay in one place longer because they no longer had to migrate when the resources of an area were exhausted. Agriculture developed to include the organized planting and harvesting of fruits, vegetables, and grains, as well as the raising of various types of livestock. This caused major shifts in the eating habits and energy profiles that had proved so beneficial to humankind up to that point.

Organized farming, and the subsequent expansion of bartering and monetary stores of value, saw the advance of specialization. Specialization allowed a goat herder to focus on his goats while the zucchini farmer could specialize in zucchinis. Specialization resulted in better rates of food production and increased value. Small villages grew into large cities and entire civilizations were born to facilitate trade. This also meant that there were all kinds of people selling all kinds of things, just as it is today, making a broader range of food choices available to more people more of the time. This, above all, has had the greatest impact on human eating habits and energy profiles.

But not all more recent developments in human eating patterns result in improved health and energy. Take, for example, the prevalence of cow's milk in the diets of people around the world. The human gastrointestinal process didn't develop to process cow's milk. Our ancient ancestors didn't stop to take the milk of other species; they didn't stop to milk a buffalo, ox, or cow. Milk didn't become a regular part of the human diet until cattle farmers began to harvest and sell everything they could from a cow, from the skin as leather, to crushed bones as fertilizer, and to milk as a beverage. This was so successful that milk, no longer an ancillary industry to the meat, became an entirely mature industry of its own. Unfortunately, no matter how much we are convinced that milk is good for us, milk is just not something that human bodies can break down and extract full benefit from. Even the calcium from milk is not fully bioavailable. One in five children in the United States have milk allergies, and that's the ones we know about. There are many more, probably as many as three in five, that have minor allergies that go unreported. Human beings didn't evolve to drink milk the milk of other species, and yet we do.

Intermittent fasting is normal
Despite changes to human eating habits over more recent history, we need to remember that human physiology originally developed under conditions that favored the consumption of certain foods and

where eating was not a daily occurrence. Human beings evolved to eat a large quantity of food, store it, and then survive on that stored energy for a few days. Once that store was depleted, humans would hunt and forage for more food. It's not just about how much we ate, it's also about how often and when we ate.

This brings us to the topic of our book, intermittent fasting. At its most basic, intermittent fasting is about when you eat, not so much about what you eat.

"Intermittent fasting" falsely conjures up an impression of difficulty and discomfort, and triggers an aversion to what is actually a natural thing for humans. We tend to see fasting as synonymous with starving, but it is not. Fasting and starving have very different clinical definitions. Fasting is when you stop using the food that you have eaten most recently as the source of energy, whereas starvation occurs when your body no longer has any stores of fat left to convert to energy and begins to convert muscle mass – in other words, the body starts attacking living tissue – to fuel essential systems. Most of us, even if we haven't eaten for a week, are nowhere near starving.

Re-evaluating our eating habits

When we begin to reconsider how we function, including the way we eat, we need to take into account three areas. The first is the machinery of the body with all its structures, tissues, and processes. The second is our brain, the seat of control and consciousness. The brain controls appetite, homeostasis, and even sleep cycles. Third is the environment around us. Not just the natural world or the air and water that sustains us, the environment is also about what we are influenced to do – the actions we mimic, the trends we follow, the culture we are a part of. Even the prevailing political climate is part of the environment that influences our health and well-being. So, in looking at intermittent fasting, we'll need to look at it from the physical and physiological standpoint, the mental standpoint, and the cultural or environmental perspective.

One of the recurring themes you'll find in this book are the role of habits in eating and fasting. Our eating habits can be like slowly accumulating toxins in more than one way. (And, as you'll see, intermittent fasting can help clear that up.)

Let me illustrate this point. If you eat enough of something toxic all at once, you will experience observable repercussions. But if you take the same thing over a long period, and in small enough quantities, you will find that the amounts you ingest that don't exceed the threshold will accumulate instead and have a long-lasting effect on our system which only becomes apparent much later. This is true of arsenic. And it is true of drinking mercury in water.

If arsenic, which is one of the most toxic and lethal substances known to man, can accumulate in the body long before it kills you, then you need to realize that the issue of habit – something that you do repeatedly, and which applies equally to what you eat – can have a significant impact on your life over time.

Human beings are creatures of habit. Once we start a habit it's hard to let go of our personal habits. There are also powerful societal habits, things we do just because that is what everyone around us does. Societal habits can include what we eat, where and when we eat it. Food habits can be based on cultural aspects of food that no longer make sense anymore for changing energy profiles and circumstances.

For example, the Inuit tribes of North America have always hunted whales as part of their diet. Two of the most prized sections of the whale are its skin and blubber, the fat just below the skin. The meat is edible, of course, and is used widely in dishes and recipes. The fat is enjoyed and accepted because it provides a huge amount of energy, fueling the Inuit's metabolism and layering their bodies with the fat necessary to battle the frigid temperatures of the Arctic. However, if an Inuit moves to more temperate latitude along the equator, he couldn't possibly continue eating a diet rich in whale blubber and would find himself battling an old habit that would be trying to override his appetite for something different and more appropriate to eat.

Eating habits and three meals a day

Habits can become established mindsets and biases that aren't supported by real understanding. One such habit is the common belief in the need to eat three square meals a day. There is nothing in our genetic makeup that requires us to eat three meals at predetermined times regardless of our lifestyle. Why would one person who works with heavy physical exertion, lifting large boxes, eat the same amount and on the same schedule as the man who sits at a desk all day watching camera monitors? Their energy requirements and overall profiles are obviously very different. There is a lot more energy expended by the delivery guy doing physical carrying and pushing than there is by a building security specialist at his desk monitoring camera feeds. One could burn 3,000 calories a day, while the other burns just 1,000. Why would it make sense that they both eat a 1,200 calorie lunch? It doesn't. The strenuously active person needs to consume significantly more calories, three times more to be exact.

Eat *what* you need *when* you need it

Each of us has a different energy profile, so it only makes sense that we should all have different consumption patterns. These consumption patterns include optimal timing and the calories required. In intermittent fasting programs, you don't need to worry too much about calories, but your goal should be to find your optimal schedule and frequency of meals. Later, we'll talk about different eating schedules and how to better understand what your appetite is telling you to eat.

Intermittent fasting is not something you will need to follow strictly for the rest of your life. You should practice it until it becomes a habit or a lifestyle. Once you get to that point, eating what you need, when you need it, will be as normal as brushing your teeth. Of course, you can always go back to a period of scheduled intermittent fasting when you want to get your systems back on track.

Although your basic practice of intermittent fasting will be to eat within certain "windows" of time, eating with less frequency, this program also suggests that you need to be eating the right foods. However, it doesn't dictate what those foods are. No one can tell you what the "right" food to eat should be. Only your own body can tell you that, and that is what you want to learn to listen to. The key here is to listen to your own appetite, and then go with it.

Although intermittent fasting is fundamentally about when you eat rather than about what you eat, if you also pay attention to what you eat, you can supercharge your systems – both the gastrointestinal and metabolic systems and their processes – into an even more finely tuned engine with a more beneficial energy profile.

During induction week, there will be a few things that you can do to help your body be better able to tell you exactly what it needs. Then, you will be able to provide your body with exactly the nutrients it is looking for without consuming unnecessary calories.

Appetite Alerts and Cravings

This brings me to the next point of taste and appetite. Your body is a highly complex organism with multiple systems interacting with each other. When you go about your daily routine, the tasks you do cause wear and tear on your systems. It's like a car. You have engine oil in the crankcase to keep the bearings and moving parts lubricated, but once in a while oil levels get too low, and a little light illuminates on the dashboard to tell you that you that the car is low on oil. Then, you need to change the oil or top it up – or, eventually, the car will develop bigger problems.

In the same way, there are many different substances, such as water, that your body needs to perform a broad variety of interactions and processes. Metabolism, for instance, is more efficient when there is sufficient hydration to perform the Krebs Cycle (the sequence of reactions by which most cells release stored energy). Your body sends you an alert when your hydration levels are low by making you feel thirsty. Thirst is an alert for dehydration. If you ignore it, you run the risk of problems that can get much worse.

This can also happen when you run out of a specific minerals or nutrients – let's say iron, as a familiar example. When you run out of this nutrient, your body tries to give you a heads-up on what it needs, and you feel a sensation or an appetite or impulse to eat things like steak or other foods high in iron. In my own case, it manifests as the desire to have a steak; my wife will suddenly have a desire to eat scallops or clams. We all have different libraries of accumulated knowledge in our body to tell us which foods have been experienced as the best sources for specific nutrients. That "library" is something we build up over the course of our lives, and is based on the foods that we have gone out in the world and tried.

Unfortunately, recent generations face a major problem in making food choices. Their senses and appetites have been trained to point them in the wrong directions. If we have become generationally incapable of choosing the right foods, then how can we be expected to make the right choices?

The battle is really between opposing impulses from your brain/body. Your brain/body knows how to trigger your sense of thirst when you need more water. In the same way, it knows how to trigger your appetite for iron-rich foods when that need arises. At the same time, however, there is another part of your brain that is craving for a "fix," the kind of fix it gets whenever you eat junk food.

So, just what is "junk food"?

Junk food is anything that is engineered for taste but is deficient in nutrition.

Sugar cravings

Take, for instance, a tablespoon of normal table sugar. It is an amazing ingredient, convenient, cheap, and pleasing. The sweetness gives you a boost of glucose. But it has zero nutrients. All the nutrients the sugar had when it was first harvested from the cane or the beet have been stripped and bleached away to produce plain sugar. Processed white sugar gets addicting very fast. Just a little and the body's surge of energy is recorded in your biological library. A few more hits of sugar and the corresponding boost in energy is an established relationship. So, the next time you need energy, you are going to crave sugar. Have you ever been in a situation where you were stressed and you started to crave candy? When the body is under stress, it craves energy to prepare for fight or flight, and if those energy stores are depleted, you need to have something sweet to replenish it fast.

Salt cravings

Salt is something else your body naturally craves. Salt is a critical ingredient in the human body, maintaining the required salinity to aid in healthy diffusion and to keep the body's electrical conductivity at its peak.

If you want to understand the role of salt in the body's electrical conductivity, try this experiment when you get a chance. Take a pail of pure water. Put a battery beside the pail, and connect a wire from the negative lead to the positive terminal of lightbulb on the other side of the pail. Connect a second wire to the positive lead of the battery, dropping the other end into the water. Connect a third wire to the negative terminal of the lightbulb and drop the other end into the water. Now you have a positive lead from the battery in the water and a negative lead from the bulb in the water, but they aren't touching. What happens? Nothing.

Now, start adding a little salt and dissolve it in the water. You won't see any difference at first because there is too little salt, but as you keep adding more, you will gradually start to see the bulb light up. This happens because salt is an electrolyte, which increases the conductivity of water, and which, in turn, allows electrons to pass, completing the electrical circuit.

There are many electrical systems in your body — your heart is one of them. The impulses that run along your nerves from your brain to the rest of your body are also electrical in nature. All of these electrical systems need salt to function. For this and other reasons, salt is constantly craved by your body, and you are rewarded when you consume it. Many junk foods take advantage of the body's natural desire for salt.

Fat cravings

The third element the body craves almost as much as sugar is fat. Think of bacon, greasy fries, or moist roasts. Fat is something that the body rewards you for when you consume it. Later on, we'll be talking about why your body rewards you for eating fat.

So, let's take a closer look at the reasons for the body's desire to consume fat, bacon, chocolates, butter, and so on. Think back to our Paleolithic ancestors and consider what their basic patterns of consumption were and how their metabolism worked. They survived on a higher ratio of fat to carbohydrates than we do today. The largest part of their meal consisted of the meat that they hunted, and they gorged on that meat. Once that was done, and they had none left, they rested and hung around their dwellings. For the next 24 to 48 hours, they didn't hunt. If they felt the need, they would pick on berries and fruits. The ratio of protein and fat to carbs that they lived on was heavily in favor of the fat and proteins, which gave them tremendous energy and mental acuity. Our ancestors had so much energy that they could chase prey, and while they couldn't always catch them, they could keep on the chase until the prey was so exhausted it would give up or die from exhaustion.

It also gave them highly tuned instincts of what to eat, and they only ate when they were hungry or when there was an opportunity.

Fat was the energy store of choice, and it was also the preferred item on the menu. The metabolic chemistry of those early humans was very different than what we have today. While the underlying systems remain the same, we are forcing it to adapt to a different environment.

Our ancestors would eventually consume this fat, and when that fat was processed in the gut and transported to all areas around the body, hours after the meal, these hunter-gatherers slept and relaxed because their body was busy stocking up on the fuel source. About 1,000-1,400 calories would be stored as glycogen in the liver and skeletal muscles, while the rest was converted to fat in a process called lipogenesis.

During lipogenesis, excess calories are converted into triglycerides and carried via the bloodstream to be deposited in different areas. At that time, this was the primary source of energy. Carbohydrates was a backup source of energy and was used for the body's functions during the time the body was processing the food. It was also used to sustain the body while the food was converted to fat.

These hunter-gatherers lived a feast-or-famine lifestyle, so the body, which relied more on fat, had to also develop a parallel system of energy creation which was dependent on fast energy from carbs and proteins. Carbs and shorter chain sugars from fruits provided an instant pick-me-up for those who were feeling lethargic, but it would be a short-lived burst of energy. The sugars would be quickly mopped up and stored as fat or flushed out of the system. Nonetheless, it was a quick access to energy.

Once the lipogenesis process was complete, people could then go about their day and do what they had to. Once they had burned through their calories and were accessing their fat stores, they would be back to feeling hungry and went off on a hunt once again.

Habit-forming dopamine "hits"

Our ancestor's energy needs were primarily driven by fats, and so, even today, when we taste fat, we are rewarded with bliss.

We like these flavors because dopamine is released whenever we have foods that are engineered just right. Unfortunately, that dopamine release can go on to do something more insidious. Because dopamine release gives pleasure, that helps to create a habit. If you do something a few times and are rewarded for it each time, it becomes a habit. Eventually, you no longer have to think about it because it has become an automatic and habitual response.

The magic triumvirate

The triumvirate of ingredients, fat, salt, and sugar, are the magic ingredients of any manufactured or processed food. Major food manufacturers spend millions to research the best mix with just the right ratio of fat, sugar and salt to get the most people "hooked" on their products. Be it potato chips, sauces, candy bars, power drinks, soda, burgers, fast foods, or any other fast or processed food, the key is to get the consumer to come back for more. They do it by playing around with the flavor, especially combinations of fat, sugar, and salt, which are naturally powerfully attractive to humans and very addictive.

The first time you consume this deliciously-engineered food, the body gets its salt, sugar, and fat, and you are rewarded with a hit of dopamine. You like the reward of feeling great after eating the food, and so you try to repeat it, and you are rewarded again. A few more times, and you are hooked. Of course, everyone has the right to choose what they put into themselves – but just because mercury is freely available doesn't mean you should ingest it.

The silencing of true cravings

Not only do these "junk" food addictions steer you toward specific food items, but they also do something else much more insidious – they silence the true appetite cravings one might otherwise have. When you can't tell what your body is craving, you can't give it what it needs.

The more you eat the foods you are addicted to, the less the chance that you are getting the nutrients you really need, and so you feel hungry more often, and end up consuming more calories, and you can end up piling on the weight.

How does this really work? Well, when it's 'time' to have a meal, the first problem is that your body alerts you by giving you a sensation that it is hungry. That's typically not the right place to start from, because your body should only get hungry when it has no energy left in reserves. And unfortunately, when your senses are clouded, you are likely to crave the usual triumvirate of salt, sugar, and fat – in some form. And that is the problem.

Even when you may not need the calories (energy), hunger can be triggered by the body's nutritional needs. If, for example, your body needs potassium, and it is urgent, then, no matter how much you feed yourself, as long as that potassium (or some other mineral) is lacking, the body will keep sending you signals of being hungry. So, you run to the pantry to make a midnight snack, or head out to an all-night diner to satisfy that hunger. Whatever you do, you have just taken on extra calories, but are probably not any closer to getting the nutrients you actually need.

This is the core reason for the prevalence of obesity in America today. Even though that obesity is easily explained away as the result of the high fat content of fast food, and so on, the real reason isn't only that we overeat, it's also that we don't get the nutrients the body really needs so our hunger is never really satisfied.

The rest of this book is devoted to looking at how you can get rid of those addictive cravings. This is an advanced version of the intermittent fast, and, more importantly, it's a strategy to get healthier, not just slimmer. Eventually, it is possible to reach the stage where the body will only give you the appetite for what needs replenishing, whether that's energy or nutrients.

Chapter 2: Overview of the Intermittent Fast

Intermittent fasting returns you to the eating patterns of the generations that influenced your genetic makeup. That genetic inheritance established the forms of human metabolic functioning and set the order of energy creation.

Metabolism of Sugars and Fats

First, there is the metabolism of sugars through the process of glycolysis to create ATP, the molecule that stores and transports energy within cells. In glycolysis, one molecule of glucose is converted into carbon dioxide and two ATP molecules in the cytoplasm of a cell. The ATP is then used as energy in the cell for whatever it needs to do. Each molecule of glucose results in 2 ATP.

Second, there is the metabolism of fats, that is, the conversion of triglycerides, a type of fat (lipid) found in the blood and stored in fat cells. The conversion of One triglyceride molecule produces 406 ATP – more than 200 times the amount of ATP generated in glycolysis. This is one advantage of burning fat for energy instead of glucose.

When you are in a perpetual intermittent fast, your body is going to gradually switch to using triglycerides instead of glucose for energy more often.

Long distance runners are experts at achieving this switch from burning glucose to burning fats. They load up on food for days before a long-distance event, and then eat right before the event, filling up their reserves of glycogen. That glycogen in the liver and skeletal muscles amounts to about 1,000-1,400 calories. Long distance runners will burn through this fast once the marathon starts. A little later, when they have exhausted all their glycogen reserves, they will begin to burn fat. People who aren't used to this will feel an immense lethargy at the point the glycogen runs out. Some will even pass out. Seasoned pros, however, know how to get past "the wall."

Once the body starts converting triglycerides, there is a short lag, but the release of energy soon speeds up as it is more efficient than converting glucose. Once the metabolism has completely switched from the metabolism of glycogen to the metabolism of triglycerides, energy becomes abundantly available. The brain is then fed with ketones, instead of glucose, while the body starts to burn fat rapidly and effectively. The runner is then back up to speed, and can run extreme distances without stopping. The only thing they need is to constantly replenish their hydration. Without the necessary hydration, those metabolic processes will stall.

Easing into Intermittent Fasting

Just as you wouldn't expect to successfully start running extreme distances overnight, you can't really jump into intermittent fasting and hope to enjoy the benefits or the process right way. It is too much of a shock to the system, and there would be a system-wide revolt. This revolt manifests itself as headaches, mood swings, and lethargy. The better way is to ease into intermittent fasting. That is the reason for having a transitional induction week.

During induction week, the objective is to get your body ready for the process of shifting from relying on glucose and glycogen stores for all your energy needs into burning fat for energy. Do not take this lightly. Restoring your body's natural metabolic processes is supposed to be great, but if you do it too abruptly, at worst, it will mess with you unpredictably, or, at best, it is going to be so uncomfortable that you will give up and quit.

Once you have spent a week (or two weeks, if you need it) making the transition of induction week, you can move onto the initial fasting period. Not only will this free up a lot of your time normally spent eating and processing food, it will set you up for eating on a schedule that suits you or gets you into the rhythm of eating only when you genuinely need to.

Finally, you will get to the maintenance part of the diet. That is when you get your body off a rigid feeding schedules to arrive at your own schedule where you can confidently listen to your own body about when to eat. That will also be when you will figure out how much to eat, and what your appetites mean, so that you will know what you are really craving.

The next chapter is all about getting prepared for intermittent fasting during your induction week. We will look at the objectives that you have to set for yourself in both physical and psychological terms as well as the logistics of it. We will also look at establishing some good new habits and abandoning some bad ones, so that you can magnify the results of your intermittent fasting.

If you are ready, it is time to get started.

Chapter 3: Induction Week

Decide when you want to begin induction week – it should take you seven straight days. In my experience, going away for the weekend is a great time to get started, because it gets you away from things you tend to do by habit. If you try to start intermittent fasting surrounded by memory stimuli, such as your dining room and kitchen, then you will be constantly reminded to grab lunch or dinner at specific times, or to go back for snacks and junk food (assuming you are a snack lover).

The point of this first week is to expand your range of gastronomical choices and to cleanse the bodily systems that can make it harder to be on an intermittent fast.

The first thing you need to do this week is to remove all the processed foods from your diet, especially the fast foods, soda, and anything that comes pre-packaged or pre-seasoned. Your best bet is to eat fresh, organic food, but if you can't get organic food, don't worry, just make sure it's fresh. Otherwise, you can eat anything you want – steaks, dairy, fish, meat. It's all fair game here.

Day 0

On Day 0, you can really eat almost anything you want, whenever you want, with a few restrictions that will start cleansing your system. On Day 0, you want to cut out caffeine, soda, processed foods, junk food, fast foods, processed salt (you can substitute sea salt or Himalayan salt), and all sugar, and candy.

Also, drink fresh water throughout the day. Mineral water is fine but avoid reverse osmosis water which losses beneficial minerals and tends to be more acidic. Add two slices of lemon to a liter of water and drink that. When you have finished the first liter, use another two slices of lemon to a fresh bottle. In total, you are going to drink 2 liters of water.

Your last meal before starting the induction week of intermittent fasting will be on the evening of Day 0.

Stop eating at 7 p.m. on Day 0, but keep your water near you. If you finish your daily quota of 2 L of water, but you still feel like drinking more, go ahead. At night, however, the water you keep next to you should just be plain and clear water. You don't need to add the two slices of lemon to your nighttime water.

Day 1

On Day 1, you are going to perform a dawn-to-dusk fast where you don't eat anything and only consume water. Fill your water bottle again with water and lemon.

Go for a walk in the morning, and see the sights of wherever you are visiting for these first days of induction week. When you feel hungry, take a sip of water, but go out and take part in any activity that does not involve eating. Go have a blast – and forget about food.

One of the goals of Day 1 is to begin resetting your mental frameworks for the way you think about food, and for when you think of food. Everything about fasting and the habits of eating are more about mental issues than they are about physical or physiological ones. Your body is not going to crave food as much as your mind is.

Continue drinking water throughout the day until 7 p.m. when you will be having supper, your one meal of the day.

Ideally, you should arrive wherever you are going to have dinner a half hour early. Since you will be breaking fast at 7 p.m., get there at 6:30 and spend some time with your thoughts. Think over the day and how often you felt hunger and what exactly that was about. Feel free to make all the notes you need. Take these moments for evaluation because you need to become more sensitive to what your cravings and appetite signals are really telling you.

For dinner, start with some juice to stimulate your appetite and digestion. You can really have just about anything you want – just stay away from the processed and junk foods. At the end of your meal, you can even treat yourself to coffee and even ice cream – so long as it is not processed. Eat as much as you want, but make sure you are listening to your stomach (you know what I mean) instead of listening to your taste buds.

Feel the food, chew it, and savor the flavors. Separate the taste of the main ingredients from the spices. Get to know your food and take your time. Have the salad, have the meat or fish, whatever you want, and, with each item, make a mental note of how much you enjoy the food.

When you are done, realize that everything is really going well. You should be proud of yourself at this point. You have overcome your usual cravings and your body, no matter how weak you felt just before you broke fast, you were doing fine.

For the rest of the day, there are no more snacks to have or beverages to drink except water. When you go to bed, keep the bottle of water by your bedside.

Day 2
When you wake up on Day 2, start with your lemon water. Whether you decide to stay in, go out on the town, or get ready to head back for the work week ahead, remember you won't be eating anything during the day.

One of the things you will want to do is to prepare for breaking your fast at home. If you can, try to make dinner at home, or at least eat at home. If you don't have the supplies, the natural or unprocessed ingredients, you'll need to stock your pantry before you cook Day 2's meal. You don't really need to fill up your house with organic ingredients (If you can, that's great, but that can be expensive).

Remember, what's most important in intermittent fasting is the schedule of eating that you keep to. But you do want to drain your system of the chemicals typically found in processed foods, because that will help you enormously with intermittent fasting.

Cleansing the System of "Junk" Foods

There are sections of recipes and lists of foods scattered throughout this book to help you get started. The objective is to expand your "library" of nutritional sources, and to remove the hold that unhealthy ingredients in processed foods have on your habits and gastronomical pleasure centers. Most people do not fully appreciate just how many of their food choices are made "under the influence" of the choices that processed foods have predisposed them to. It's like giving a kid candy – after a while, that's all they want to eat because that candy has predisposed them to a sugary diet. In a similar way, processed foods predispose you to an unhealthy and inadequate diet.

Induction week is all about returning freedom of choice to you. Once you get rid of the toxins from your diet, they become less of a distraction as you move forward with intermittent fasting. Without the transition of the induction phase of the program, when you try to expand your food choices, the intermittent fast will become very difficult because of the addictions to salt, sugar, and fat and all the other ingredients in typical processed items, such as nitrates, hydrogenated oils, high fructose corn syrup, and flavor enhancers.

The focus of induction week is on cleansing the body of those habits and on flushing your system out as your body is rebalanced in the absence of the accumulated toxins. This will do two things for you. First, it stops the cravings for food when you are not really hungry. Second, it changes the kinds of food you crave, allowing you to have an appetite only for what your body actually needs.

Just be aware, the effort to remove the addiction to processed foods will be a tough one. But that is exactly what you need to do to make sure that you regain control and the power of choice. It is not that simple to scrub your addiction to a particular item. There are many ways to overcome an addiction, whether to nicotine, alcohol, opioids, food items, or anything else, but they are not always the same way, because the chemistry of addiction varies by substance. The severity of each addiction also differs, and therefore its hold and what it takes to overcome will also differ.

The addiction to processed foods can be severe, at best. Food is a matter of life and death and the brain sees the lack of it as a threat to existence. And even more in the modern world is the idea of stopping food simply scorned. However, fasting for a day overcomes this fallacy, and serves to cleanse the chemical echoes that cause the difficulty.

Caloric needs and addictive cycles

All of your food intake will fall into one of two categories: first, what satisfies your caloric needs for the day, and, second, what satisfies the nutritional needs of the day.

Caloric needs are those needs you have for the energy all cells need to function. Without energy, nothing works. For this reason, the brain is designed to seek out energy and to calculate how much energy it needs. The brain sees taking in calories as the ultimate security feature. Without energy, the brain becomes dysfunctional and then the body dies. Because it is so important, any time energy is given to the body, you are rewarded with a rush of dopamine, and that, in turn, creates a habit. Children are especially susceptible to this habit-forming cycle, because they need loads of energy to fuel their activities and growth, yet they have a small gastrointestinal capacity.

PH balance, digestion and nutrients

Adding lemon to your drinking water starts to change the acidity of your internal chemistry. Not only does the lemon help maintain your body's electrolyte balance, but lemon is an incredible fruit with unconventional acid-alkaline properties. Usually, when you ingest something acidic, like vinegar, it enters your system and remains acidic. It has an acidic bias in your blood chemistry. That makes sense – if it is acidic outside, it's acidic inside. But this is not so with the lemon you add to your drinking water. Lemon has the uncanny ability to change from acid to alkaline once it is digested in the body. It's net effect on your digestive system and then your blood is to make it mildly alkaline.

The human body, itself, has a variety of pH profiles. Acid levels in the stomach, for instance, are between 2 and 3.5 pH. This is the reason you have a mucosal layer to protect the tissues of the stomach from erosion by the acids secreted during the digestive process. When the digested food (called chyme) leaves the stomach, it is highly acidic at about 2 pH, and that is not a good thing for the digestive tract. The digestive tract is a porous sheath that allows water to carry the released nutrients across its membrane to the network of blood vessels that encapsulates its entire length. To counter the inhospitable acidity, the duodenum releases *cholecystokinin*, a hormone that signals the gallbladder to reduce the acidity by releasing bile which is highly alkaline. By the time the chyme passes to the rest of the small intestine, it is at a neutral or even slightly alkaline pH. That permits efficient absorption of nutrients across the membrane and into the blood.

One side effect of eating processed foods is to raise acid levels in the body. The few days you stop eating the heavily processed foods that cause acid-forming substances to accumulate, while drinking lemon water to counteract the acidity of the digestive environment, will make a huge difference in the way your body functions, and how effectively nutrients are absorbed.

Nutrition density vs. calories

The more effectively you absorb the nutrients your body needs, the less calories (energy) you will need to ingest. Remember the duality of all the foods we consume – calories versus nutrients. Let's be clearer about that. Everything you ingest has calories. Even if you chewed paper up and swallowed it, it will have a caloric value. Whether you eat beef to get the iron you need, or eat salmon, aside from the taste, the difference lies in the number of calories you take in as you get your iron. This is referred to as nutrition density. On the one hand, substances like table sugar have zero nutrition but a high number of calories. On the other hand, foods like broccoli have lots of nutrients and low calories.

Processed foods that create addictive cycles are low ratio items, meaning that they have high amounts of calories but low levels of nutrients. So, while you get more than the amount of energy you need for the day, you aren't getting enough of the nutrients, micronutrients, and vitamins the body needs to replenish itself. Energy is just one part of the equation. All the energy in the world is not going to help you pedal a bicycle if your muscles are not functioning properly as the result improper tissue maintenance caused by a lack of the right nutrients.

The following is a list of examples of foods that have a high nutrient density. You should try to include as many of these kinds of foods as you can during the induction period.

- Beef Liver

- Salmon

- Broccoli

- Kale

- Shellfish

- Potatoes

- Sardines

- Garlic

- Seaweed

- Dark Chocolate

You want to start resetting your body's "library" of food choices to include foods with a high nutrition density so that you take in the greatest amount of nutrients for the least number of calories. Given the opportunity, your body can start recognizing and craving nutrient rich foods. You are certainly not required to eat these foods exclusively, but eating more nutrient dense food, in itself, will begin to help you drop any unwanted weight.

How unsatisfied nutritional hunger piles on calories

Let's look at the way that unsatisfied cravings for nutrients can cause you to eat more calories than you need.

Let's say your body is telling you that it is hungry and that you have an appetite for beef liver, something in your body's nutrient "library." There is a good chance that something like iron or B-complex is in deficit in your body – which is normal – it just needs to be replenished. But instead of frying up some liver, you decide to reach for that extra-large slice of cheesecake. Initially, it fills you up, you feel good, and you have taken on 400 calories. Once your stomach has gone through processing that cheesecake, your system recognizes that the nutrients it needs are still not there, so it sends another signal to your brain that it needs liver, but you still don't give it liver. Instead, you fill up on a peanut butter sandwich. There's another 150 calories. Now you are up to 550 calories, and your body still hasn't received what it has been asking for.

By this point, you're very hungry, so you head over to your favorite diner, and finally have that plate of liver and onions. It hits the spot, but you now have added another 400 calories. You are no longer hungry, but you've taken on a total of 950 calories. If you had just listened to your body, and got what it was asking for all along, you wouldn't have eaten that extra 550 calories. Extrapolate this pattern out over a week, or an entire year, and you can easily see why two out of three North American adults are either overweight or obese.

There are all sorts of diets that don't account for the body's nutritional requirements and focus only on calories. This is counterproductive, both for losing the excess weight, and for being healthy.

Intermittent fasting is about changing the frequency of your meals to suit your metabolic profile. However, by also paying attention to your nutritional needs, you can learn to let your body to tell you when it is hungry only when it has real nutritional needs, instead of piling on calories that are beyond what it needs for energy.

Processed foods vs. your body's "library" of nutritional sources

Processed foods also diminish the efficacy of the intermittent fast in another way. Suppose you ate a fast food burger, taking in all the salt, sugar and fat that went with it, and you feel good. The problem is that it is nutritionally deficient, right? Yes, but it is worse than that.

That burger does have some nutrition, so the body records this food item in its "library" as a possible source for the nutrients it needs. So, let's say a fast food burger supplies 20% of your daily B12 requirement but also supplies 400 calories – you would need five burgers to reach that daily B12 requirement. That's 2,000 calories that you would have to take in. Compare that to a fresh serving of lightly grilled salmon that is only about 250 calories yet supplies 100% of your daily B12 requirement.

If you only expose yourself to fast food burgers, your body will believe that the burger is the only source of B12, so every time you need B12, your cravings will direct you to that fast food burger. However, when you introduce a great tasting freshly grilled and nutrient-packed salmon, especially during induction week when you have stopped all processed food, your body will begin to update the records in its nutritional "library," especially after a number of repetitions of the experience. Eventually when you need B12, you'll experience a hankering for grilled salmon, instead of the burger with its unnecessary extra calories.

Summary of Goals for Induction Week

During this intermittent fasting program, the objectives of induction week are to:

- Ease the addictive hold of processed foods,

- Increase the variety of fresh foods in your diet,

- Improve the nutritional density of your food,

- Improve the alkaline/acid balance of your body, and

- Drink plenty of water.

Day 3

On Day 3, you are probably back at work after your weekend, and you should start your day with a brisk walk. An average of a 30-minute walk around the block is a great way to start your day. The increased metabolism from walking and the increased oxygen intake from the fresh morning air will go a long way toward getting your metabolism working.

Turning fat-burning metabolism "on"

At this point, it won't be your regular metabolism — the one that burns glucose and glycogen — that is kicking into gear, it will be the metabolism that uses triglycerides. That means you will be burning fat. Once you start burning fat, every minute of workout you do has an impact on your weight loss objective or at least contributes to your overall effort.

The average person burns about 1,800 to 2,200 calories per day (women) and 2,800 to 3,200 calories per day (men). Those ranges take into account overall lifestyle. The higher calorie burn numbers are for those with active lifestyles, and the lower numbers are for those who are less active.

When you sleep, you burn about 0.42 calories per pound of body weight per hour of sleep. So, let's say you are 180 pounds and sleep 8 hours a night. You can calculate that by multiplying 0.42 by your weight in pounds by the number of hours you sleep. In this example, that would work out as 0.42 x 180 x 8 or 605 calories. That's just when you sleep.

When you wake up and go out for your 30-minute walk in the morning, you are going to burn approximately 200 calories. By the time you hit the showers in the morning, you have already used up 800 calories. Remember that your body only stores about 1,400 calories in the liver and the skeletal muscles. Once that has been used up, the body will have to switch metabolic engines and begin to burn fat stores instead.

When you get to work, even if you are sitting all day, you are burning about 70 calories per hour. Over the entire day, that's 700 calories (on the low side). So, now, you are already up to about 1,500 calories, past the body's glycogen stores (unless you consume food along the way). That means you will come to a point where you feel tired, and then, a little while later, you will feel an energy surge as the triglycerides start being converted for energy. Once you start burning fat for energy, you will notice how powerful and alert you feel.

Although the body does well burning fat as fuel, it can't do it all on fat-based energy. You are not limiting your food sources, except for avoiding refined sugar and processed food. When you eat anything you feel like, you will find that you end up getting any carbohydrates you need as well as the nutrients. The carbohydrates you take in will provide the glucose the brain needs, which is about 20% of total fuel. If you can feed your brain that ratio of 80:20, you will start to see an uptick in mental performance.

During induction week, you are getting your body to experiment with repeated switching between fuel sources. Your body has been accustomed to using glucose and glycogen as its primary energy source. In the beginning, fasting will feel hard, because your body has forgotten how to switch from glycogen to triglycerides. But it will remember when it is pushed. You just have to hold fast.

During induction week, you will have triggered triglyceride metabolism at least once every day, and that will create a visceral memory of how to do it at a moment's notice. It will also fine-tune the process so that it triggers and stabilizes faster. By the time you get to intermediate week, your body should have become more proficient at making the change quickly. It won't be perfect, but it will be getting there.

Days 3 to 7

For days 3 to 7, the schedule will stay the same through the rest of the week.

Every day, go for that brisk walk in the morning, for about 30 minutes. If you have a treadmill, that's great, but try to get out to breathe the fresh morning air. It really does make a difference.

You won't eat anything throughout the day, so at lunchtime, if you are in an office or other work environment, try to politely excuse yourself from the lunch crowd, and go to the park or a museum instead. If you have the energy, go to the gym. But whatever you do, stay away from friends who are eating. The idea is to keep your mind off of food and the usual schedule for eating. You have a deeply entrenched habit of eating at lunchtime. You need to jettison that habit and being around people who are eating lunch is not going to help.

Later, when you get home, you can eat almost anything you want to, but stick to these simple guidelines:

1.   No processed food or ingredients,

2.   No sugar, and

3.   No fast foods.

Keep drinkable water with a slice of lemon with you at all times. Take a sip anytime you feel a little dry in the mouth, or you think you feel hungry.

One of the things you will notice is that your urine will become clear after the second or third day. Proper hydration, plus a little bit more, will be helping to flush accumulated toxins, and the electrolytes from the lemon will balance the salinity of the systems in your body.

At the end of this transitional induction week, evaluate whether you need to go a day or more than the seven days that you have already done. How would you know? That will vary from one person to the next. If you have found it getting easier for you to stick to one meal a day, it means your body has started to get the proper nutrients, and that your metabolism has become more adaptable. If you feel this is true, then it will be time to move on to the next phase, intermediate week.

12 Recipes

The following are some recipes to inspire you to the kind of eating you want to take you through induction week. You aren't required to eat these foods. These recipes are only provided here to make it easier for you. This is not like some other diets where the routine is fixed.

Whatever you eat, keep the ingredients fresh and unprocessed. This will help flush your system of toxins and chemicals while adding to your body's personal "library" of foods that do your body good. Once your body starts to feel really good, it will begin to prefer this type of food over others, and your body will like the feeling of staying light and active with the new eating schedule.

Grilled Salmon

2 lbs. (900 g) side of salmon (skin on)

½ teaspoon fine sea/Himalayan salt

½ teaspoon ground black pepper

8 teaspoons extra virgin olive oil

3 teaspoons mixed fresh herbs (tarragon, marjoram, thyme, and parsley), chopped

olive oil

juice of 3 lemons

Clean salmon with cool running water. Pat dry. Rub the sea salt into the fish and wrap with three layers of clean disposable kitchen towels. This will extract the moisture from the salmon. Set aside for 10 minutes.

Using a mortar and pestle, grind the herbs, pepper, and olive oil into a runny paste.

Remove the disposable towels from the salmon, leaving the salt that has stuck to the fish. Using your hands, rub the oil/pepper/herb paste all over the salmon.

Use additional olive oil to grease a heated grill. Cook the salmon on the grill for about 15 minutes. You only need to flip it once or three times.

Drizzle salmon with lemon juice before serving.

Yield: 8 servings

Beetroot Feta Salad

2 oz. (60 g) cooked beetroot, cubed

1 oz. (30 g) feta cheese, cubed

2 oz. (60 g) spinach, blanched

lemon

sea salt

ground black pepper

Toss beetroot, feta cheese, and spinach together. Squeeze the lemon over it. Add sea salt and pepper to taste.

Yield: 1 serving

Mexican Sausage Delight

1 Mexican chorizo sausage (2.8 oz.) (80 g)

2 Italian sausages (2.8 oz.) (80 g)

2 large eggs

1 small red onion, diced

1 jalapeno pepper, chopped

1 teaspoon paprika

3 tablespoons extra virgin olive oil

juice from 1 fresh lime

juice from 1 fresh lemon

juice from 3 fresh calamondin lime

sea salt

ground black pepper

1 teaspoon fresh oregano

1 cup cherry tomatoes, quartered

1 red bell pepper, chopped

1 medium spring onion, chopped

1 large avocado, diced

2 teaspoons fresh coriander

sour cream

Poach eggs in boiling salted water. Use a slotted spoon to remove the eggs from the water. Set the eggs aside on a kitchen towel to absorb excess water. Season the eggs with sea salt and pepper to taste.

De-case the sausages and fry the meat in a dry pan until the meat browns and cooks. It should take no longer than 6 minutes. Add the red onions and jalapenos and continue to cook, stirring until the onions soften. Sprinkle with paprika. Reduce heat to medium and continue frying until the meat turns a darker shade of brown. Remove from heat.

Combine olive oil, juices from the lemons and limes, salt, and pepper in a separate bowl. Add tomatoes, oregano, peppers, avocado, and spring onion. Toss it all together to make a simple salsa.

To serve, start with the meat and place the egg on top of it. Top all with the salsa mix, then add the sour cream and coriander.

Yield: 2 servings

Sweet Plums & Yogurt
3.5 oz. (100 g) natural yogurt

2 plums, pitted and chopped

1 tsp. of honey

Combine and serve.

Yield: 1 serving

Turkey Patties
turkey, minced

small egg, beaten

spring onion, chopped

garlic

chili powder to taste

Mix the egg in with the turkey, spring onion, garlic, and chili. Discard extra egg, if any.

Form the mixture into patties. Fry patties on a grill.

Yield: 1 serving

Roast Vegetables with Balsamic Vinegar
1 roasted zucchini (courgette)

1 roasted eggplant (aubergine)

1 roasted butternut squash

1 roasted red pepper

1 tbsp. balsamic vinegar

juice of 1 lemon

Chop and slice all.

Combine all together with the lemon juice and balsamic vinegar.

Yield: 1-2 servings

Hummus with Vegetables

1 cup hummus

carrots, chopped

cucumber, chopped

green and/or red pepper, chopped

edamame beans

rock salt

Steam vegetables and edamame. Add salt. Spoon over hummus.

Yield: 1-2 servings

Turkey Breasts & Spinach

1 turkey breast steak

1 tablespoon clarified butter

1 cup cooked spinach

sea salt

Melt butter in skillet. Fry turkey breast.

Serve turkey over bed of spinach seasoned with salt.

Yield: 1 serving

Pita Pizza Wrap
whole meal pita

Philadelphia cream cheese

1 tomato, chopped

mixed herbs

sea salt

ground black pepper

Spread cream cheese over pita. Sprinkle with tomato, herbs, salt, and pepper. Fold to serve.

Yield: 1 serving

Aioli
6 cloves fresh garlic, peeled

2 tablespoons extra virgin olive oil

dash sea salt

¼ lemon

To make aioli, blend all ingredients above in a food processor to a smooth paste. If you have a large food processor, you'll need to make more; just multiply the quantities given, keeping the ratio of ingredients as above.

Use in recipes as directed.

Aioli Chicken with Vegetable Couscous
1 chicken breast

1 tablespoon aioli paste (see above)

3.5 oz. (100 g) vegetable couscous, cooked

Coat chicken with aioli. Grill the chicken. Mound couscous on the grilled chicken, and serve.

Yield: 1 serving

Roasted Red Pepper & Chicken Soup
7 oz. (200 g) chicken, cubed

1 chicken stock cube

4 cups water

½ roasted red pepper, chopped

½ roasted tomato, chopped

½ roasted onion, chopped

1 clove garlic, chopped

1 tsp. tomato puree

½ tsp. cumin

½ tsp. balsamic vinegar

sea salt

ground black pepper

Boil the chicken and stock cube in a pot of water. Remove the chicken and set aside.

Add the rest of the ingredients to the pot. Use a stick blender to puree until smooth. Return the chicken pieces to the pot and serve.

Yield: 2 servings

Shopping List

In addition to ingredients from the recipes, you can use this as a shopping list and keep ingredients from it on standby in your pantry.

Oils

avocado oil
clarified butter (ghee)
coconut oil
cod liver oil
flax oil
olive oil

Beans, etc.

> lentils
>
> quinoa

Nuts and Seeds

> almonds
>
> cashews
>
> chestnuts
>
> pumpkin seeds
>
> sesame seeds
>
> sunflower seeds

Herbs, Spices, and Condiments

> apple cider vinegar
>
> basil
>
> bay leaves
>
> black pepper
>
> cayenne pepper
>
> cilantro
>
> cinnamon
>
> garlic
>
> ginger root
>
> parsley
>
> sea salt
>
> soy sauce
>
> umeboshi vinegar (plum vinegar)

Fruits

apples

apricots

avocados

bananas

blackberries

blueberries

cantaloupe

cherries

coconut

grapefruit

grapes

honeydew melon

lemons

limes

nectarines

olives, green

oranges

papaya

pears

peaches

persimmon

pineapple

raisins

raspberries

strawberries

tangerines

watermelon

Vegetables

artichokes

asparagus

beets

bell peppers

broccoli

brussels sprouts

cabbage

carrots

cauliflower

celery

collard greens

cucumbers

eggplant

endive

kale

kohlrabi

mushrooms

mustard greens

okra

onions

parsnips

potatoes

snow peas

string beans

summer squash

sweet potatoes

yams

winter squash

zucchini

Extras

apple juice
ginger tea
grape juice
grapefruit juice
green/herbal tea
mineral water
molasses
orange juice
pineapple juice
raw cane sugar
rice syrup
wild rice

Chapter 4: Intermediate Week

Congratulations! You have just graduated to the intermediate week of this intermittent fasting program. Those periods of fasting should have been getting easier. You really need to pat yourself on the back. This past week is a real accomplishment. You have not only put your body through a tough week, you have also trained your mind to stay strong in the face of a great challenge.

Objectives for Intermediate Week

Now, your objective will be to focus your efforts on triggering fat metabolism. That is your yardstick.

During the coming week, the objective will be to lengthen the gaps between food on some days, and to have longer pockets of time to eat rather than to fill up in one meal. This will allow you to eat smaller quantities, while your body spends less time eating and more time doing other things, such as strengthening your immune system.

The objective of this week is to shorten the cycles of switching between the energy sources. You want the body to learn to adapt to a faster process of switching to burning fat for energy. For those of you looking to lose weight, or have aesthetic motives in mind, this is good news. If you are looking to do this for mental clarity, or simply to get healthier, burning fat is also good news for you. During your intermediate week of intermittent fasting, you should start to experience some positive effects. You will feel brighter, clearer, and more alert; you will start to feel more energy; and you will start to find that you are losing weight.

The point of intermittent fasting is to get the body functioning at optimal levels and to the full potential it has evolved to. Using energy from triglycerides (fats) is like using nitrous oxide in a car. It boosts both your body and your mind. If you happen to have fat to spare from years of accumulation, you will also lose the weight and feel better for it.

But what are you going to burn once you have used up (or don't have) excess weight? That is where you start taking on a high-fat content diet. This may sound counter-intuitive to generations who have been told that fat is unhealthy. Certainly, unnatural fat is bad for you, but natural animal-based fat is good for you. If you are vegan or vegetarian, there are alternatives to animal-based fats that you can consume if you are looking to burn fat for fuel. There is a section for vegans and vegetarians later in this chapter.

Cholesterol and Intermittent Fasting

We can't really talk about deliberately eating fats without talking about cholesterol. In fact, understanding cholesterol is a key to understanding how fat metabolism works in the body and in intermittent fasting.

Practitioners of intermittent fasting are likely to see changes in their cholesterol profiles during intermediate week, so this is a good time to address the issue of cholesterol.

How is your cholesterol level? Have you had it checked recently? Are you concerned about cholesterol? Do you intentionally avoid foods that contain cholesterol? You may think that fat and cholesterol are unhealthy and will lead to coronary problems. But that isn't really an accurate picture. Before you keep going on that track, there are some things that you need to know.

First, you need to understand that your body needs cholesterol. It is a critical lipoprotein without which we would not survive. Cholesterol is needed by cells – it is what is used to make cell membranes. It is also what is used to make the protective sheath protecting your nerves. Cholesterol also aids in the production of some of the most important hormones in your body, including progesterone and estrogen. You don't even need to ingest cholesterol-rich foods to have cholesterol in your blood – your liver already makes plenty.

Lipids

A lipid is a general classification that includes different kinds of cholesterol, monoglycerides, diglycerides, triglycerides, fatty acids, and more. Lipids are biomolecules that cannot be dissolved in water or water-based liquids, including blood. Putting lipids into blood would be like pouring oil into water.

Earlier, we talked about triglycerides, a lipid, being moved through the bloodstream. Since lipids, on their own, are not water-soluble, they need to be attached to a protein to make them soluble in water – these are called lipoproteins. In other words, the lipids found in your circulatory system are floating around in the form of lipoproteins. Specifically, lipoproteins are found in your blood in five different forms of cholesterol.

5 types of cholesterol

The five types of cholesterol include the HDL and LDL forms that most people have heard of, but there are three more, including chylomicrons, VLDL and IDL. VLDL is an acronym for Very Low-Density Lipoprotein, and IDL stands for Intermediate Density Lipoprotein.

Let's look at each of them briefly.

High Density Lipoproteins (HDLs) move triglycerides to the liver for excretion. HDLs are considered good cholesterols.

Chylomicrons are made in the gastrointestinal tract. They carry the triglycerides made from the food you eat and that are being transported around the body.

After a meal, there are higher levels of chylomicrons in the blood.

Very Low-Density Lipoproteins (VLDLs) are like chylomicrons in that they also carry triglycerides. However, VLDLs are created in the liver rather than the gastrointestinal track. VLDLs are packets of lipids that circulate to tissues where they are extracted. Once the triglyceride has been extracted by the cell, what is left is called an IDL.

Intermediate Density Lipoproteins (IDLs) are what's left once the triglycerides have been extracted, in part or in full, by the adipose tissue in the cardiac, skeletal muscles, as well as the subcutaneous layer. While the chylomicrons and VLDL are at high levels after a meal, after a few hours, the IDLs are higher, once the triglycerides have been deposited at their destinations around the body.

Low-Density Lipoproteins (LDLs) were once IDLs, but, after even more lipids have been extracted from them, they are reduced to being more shell than lipid. Remember that lipoproteins are lipids wrapped in protein shells for the purpose of transporting them through an aqueous solution. In the case of LDLs, most or all of those lipids have already been deposited in tissues all over the body. LDLs are considered the "bad" cholesterols.

Metabolic Momentum and Weight Loss

You should lose more weight this week. But that will only happen if you satisfy two prerequisites. First, continue drinking the 2 liters of lemon water. Second, walk for at least 30 minutes, briskly, first thing in the morning. Do it first thing in the morning, not later, not in the evening - but in the morning. Even if you are already in the practice of going to the gym, you still need to do this walk in the morning. During induction and intermediate weeks, you can't replace the walking with going to the gym.

Momentum is one reason you start losing weight. We face momentum in everything we do. Most things that are not the subject of effort are the physical manifestations of momentum, and this applies to all aspects of life – physical or conceptual. It's just like a car that you can accelerate to 100 km/h by flooring the gas, and once at 100 km/h, you can coast at that speed using a lot less gas. Momentum is the force that carries you forward.

Weight loss occurs when you gain metabolic momentum. When you constantly rely on glucose to fuel your daily physical and mental activities, you create a metabolic momentum that is in constant search for and use of glucose. Then, when you are out of energy, when that tank is empty, you instinctively search for glucose-heavy foods. In time, that becomes a habit. Unfortunately, when the body is driven by the metabolic momentum of using glucose, it starts a series of chain events that can destroy the body.

If the body starts supplying energy using fats and proteins instead, the body becomes more efficient. There are no insulin spikes, and no possibility of insulin resistance. You can build up a metabolic momentum to burn fat for energy instead.

Of course, you will still eat some carbohydrates along the way, and that is a good thing. This is not like the Atkins diet with its strict effort to stick only to proteins and fats, and its concerns about interrupting ketosis (metabolism of burning fat). No. In this intermittent fasting approach, you do want to include some carbohydrates in your diet. You want fats and proteins too – you basically want all things in your meal – if your body calls for them. There is no exclusion of food groups. The only thing to stop completely are processed foods.

Freeing up energy for more
Part of the momentum your body is developing is to devote more energy to the other processes of living life. It is about balance; your body needs the energy to do a variety of things beyond eating.

If you spend your day eating every few hours, then, those of you who are a little more advanced in age will recognize that your body starts to slow down after a meal, perhaps even nodding off. If you are younger, you might also have this problem, but you have certainly observed it in older folks. Those in their forties and fifties typically slow down after a meal. If they don't have coffee or caffeine in any form after a meal, they may come to a grinding halt.

This occurs because it takes a lot of energy resources for the body to digest and transport nutrients across the full length and breadth of the body. Numerous processes are at work in digestion and in circulating and moving nutrients. While this is going on, other systems are intentionally slowed down. Blood is directed away from the brain and limbs toward the length of the gut to extract and absorb nutrients and to move everything around.

When we eat every few hours through the day, the body has hardly any time to do anything else. One of the most important and beneficial things the body could be doing instead of constantly dealing with digestive processes is energizing the immune system to maintain the body's defenses.

Over the last five years, I have conducted two 30-day fasts which were very different in experience and outcome. The first was not only the most fulfilling and invigorating, it was also an eye-opener. One of the things that happened was that several scars on my leg from bike accidents faded. I had expected it, having read of others experiencing that, but it was still a breathtaking experience. More research, hours of conversations with fasting practitioners, and sessions with doctors helped me to understand why those scars disappeared.

Imagine it this way: if you hire a housekeeper to cook and clean for you, there are tasks in the house that you can delegate to your helper while you go out and take care of business. If you don't eat at home on most days, this helper will have to do fewer chores related to cooking and cleaning up after meals. With the focus on keeping the home clean, you would see a lot of cleaning done. The house would be tidy and spotless. Even the smallest of issues and details, like dust on door hinges, are likely to be taken care of.

However, if you started to stay at home more, only leaving for meals, that same helper would now be spending some of their time cleaning up after you. It would add a little to their routine, but there would still be lots of time to do the regular cleaning. Some of the finer cleaning details may take a hit, but, for the most part, all would still be well.

Now let's take this a few steps further. Suppose that not only do you begin to eat at home, with your helper doing all the cooking and after-meal clean-up, but you also have started eating every few hours. By the time you have finished one meal and the helper has cleaned up after it, it's almost time to start preparing the next meal. Most of the helper's time is now spent in the kitchen or running to the store for food. How is the rest of the house going to get cleaned? At best, you are going to run the helper ragged. Some chores would certainly get shelved and not done at all, tasks would begin to pile up, dust in the crevices would build up, and the house would start to fall into disarray.

I think you can see where I am going with this. The same thing happens with the resources in your body. When your body has to manage the intake of nutrients and the processes of moving them around, other functions have to be put on hold. The body automatically directs the use of resources according to a built-in priority system. For example, digestive processes stop instantly when fight or flight alarms are activated in the body, because digestion is a less immediate survival priority. On the other hand, digestion is given priority over other functions when the body's resources are managed.

Energy to clean up LDL cholesterol
One of the other things that happened to me after my first 30-day fast was that my LDL (the bad cholesterol) levels plummeted. That and the clearing of my scars are related in a common way.

Recall that there are five major types of cholesterol, and that cholesterol is just another word for bags of fat on their way to storage sites around the body.

When you eat, glucose is released to power the body, glycogen is stored in the liver and muscles to power the body for about half a day, and the rest is converted to fat, ready for longer term storage. Those triglycerides (fats) are packaged and prepared for distribution to different areas of the body. Since triglycerides need to be packaged in a protein sheath to be soluble in blood, those protein bags act like the bags you get when you go to the grocery store. Now imagine that your bloodstream is teeming with these bags of triglycerides on their way to different destinations in the body. Once a bag arrives at a particular place, it unloads some of those triglycerides, then it moves on to another location and unloads some more.

Once the bags have been effectively emptied, they become low-density lipoproteins (LDLs), with very low amounts of lipids in the protein bag. These are like the empty plastic bags that get tossed away onto the street after use. They enter the drainage system, blocking it, causing street flooding, and other problems. In the same way, those proteins sheets remain in the blood and accumulate over time. They start to form plaque which causes hardening and congestion of the arteries.

However, if the body is not constantly digesting food and shunting energy and fats around, it can shift into clean-up and repair mode. It can repair scars and remove unrecognized or unwanted tissue, such as LDLs. That's what happened to me during my fast, as my body redirected its time and energy to restoring my system, as good as new.

Stimulating Hormones with Fasting

The body is a powerful mechanism with the ability to keep the body stable by altering various hormones and regulating mechanisms. When it comes to fasting, there are three hormones, in particular, that you should know about – cortisol, noradrenalin, and HGH (human growth hormone).

Cortisol is a hormone with multiple purposes and it is part of the cocktail of elements released by the adrenal glands when a person stops eating during intermediate fasting or extended fasting. Among other things, cortisol regulates and controls

- blood pressure,
- the use of carbs, fats, and proteins,
- inflammation,
- blood glucose, and
- the sleep cycle.

Noradrenalin is also released. It is primarily involved in maintaining the homeostasis of the body and keeping the body's balance under all circumstances. Together with cortisol, noradrenalin is involved with returning the body to normal levels. The release of noradrenalin helps with the body's ability to return itself to the way the body was designed to be. Periods of fasting kickstarts this process.

Finally, HGH, human growth hormone, is the most important for our discussion. Human growth hormone is made by the pituitary gland. Deficiencies in HGH can lead to higher body fat retention, and decreased lean body mass and reduced bone mass. Fasting triggers HGH, so fasting is one way to counter those effects.

HGH lasts mere minutes after its release before it is metabolized by the liver and broken down into other compounds and hormones. One of these is IGF1 (insulin-like growth factor 1).

In natural and regular cycles, IGF1 is released by the body 2-3 hours before your regular wake up time. This was a curious finding, but it was eventually explained as the body, which is in a habit of waking up at a certain time, preparing for a boost of energy. So, if you are usually up by 7 a.m., you will get a shot of IGF1 at around 4 a.m. This explains why breakfast isn't the necessity that myth would have it be, and why you are still able to go for the morning walk even when you are fasting.

The human growth hormone plays a huge role in the regeneration and replacement of your bones, muscles and other tissue. Stimulating HGH during consistent periods of fasting allows your body to enjoy the benefits of the hormone without becoming immune to it. HGH also has an impact on the brain, both in terms of regeneration and creation of new neurons.

Intermediate Week Plan

During intermediate week, you should plan for longer fasting gaps with 4-hour eating "windows." This means that you can eat smaller portions more frequently during those eating windows rather one large meal.

You should also start to consume more fat and protein and fewer carbohydrates in your diet.

Make sure to have between 7 to 9 hours of sleep every night. Wake up no later than 7 a.m. and get out for your morning walk. This gets your body performing at a level that is healthy, expresses necessary hormones, and allows your metabolism to peak at a level that is constantly burning energy.

Make your morning walk a brisk one. If you were doing about 4 miles per hour last week, this week up it to about 4.5 mph and increase it to 45 minutes.

During your eating "windows," you will have 4 hours to eat whatever you want, but in smaller quantities. Then stop eating until the next eating "window," consuming only water with your trusty wedge of lemon.

There are three different eating schedules during intermediate week. Each will have a significant impact on how you adapt to this new approach to energy management. During induction week, you have already fasted for seven days having just one meal a day, so adapting to this more rigorous regime should be significantly easier.

Remember that the eating "windows" are open for 4 hours, so you can arrange your eating as you see fit.

The first of the three plans, Day 1 (D1), is to have one meal in the evening after 7 p.m. Do not have any food prior to this all day. Only have the water to drink. Arrange your day so that after you have consumed your meal, you can relax for the rest of the evening and then go off to sleep.

For that evening meal, you can choose from any of recipes in this chapter. You aren't limited to those, but I urge you to look through them to see the type of food suggested. Have a full meal, and you can have one, two, or three servings.

For Day 2 (D2), do not eat at all. Only water. Continue to go for your daily walks and have a normal day. Do what you would otherwise do, but make sure that you stay away from the kitchen. We eat more with our minds than with our stomach.

On Day 3 (D3), you will not eat anything in the morning, but you will have a good lunch. You can eat as many portions as you feel – but do not overeat. Do not think that you should load up just so you can fast longer. It doesn't work that way. Eat what you can and stop when you are full. Choose whatever you feel like having – only make sure that it's not processed food or items containing sugar. You will still need to consume at least 2L of water daily. There are no other meals on D3.

Again on Day 4 (D4), you will cleanse your system by not eating anything.

On Day 5 (D5), have a good breakfast after your walk. Don't think of it as breakfast – have a full meal, two portions if you like and if your body demands it. But don't persuade yourself that you should eat more than your body really needs. Don't eat until you are stuffed. Eat what you need, then stop.

Again, don't eat anything on Day 6 (D6).

Have another lunch or afternoon meal on Day 7 (D7).

Meal	DAY						
	1	2	3	4	5	6	7
Morning	0	0	0	0	MD5	0	0
Afternoon	0	0	AD3	0	0	0	AD7
Evening	ED1	0	0	0	0	0	0

ED1 – Evening Day 1

AD3 – Afternoon Day 3

MD5 – Morning Day 5

AD7 – Afternoon Day 7

Adding Fruit to Meals

You can add a boost by having a portion of fruits with each meal or during any eating "window." The following would be ideal, but any fruit with a pH between 3 and 4.5 works well.

Fruit	Glycemic Index	pH
Apples	39	3.6
Cherries	20	4.3
Dried Apricot	32	3.3
Grapefruit	25	3.5
Grapes	53	3
Peaches	42	3.5
Pears	38	4
Strawberries	41	3.5

Although fruits (and vegetables) may have an acidic pH to start with, they will actually help to balance a lot of the foods that are on your meal plan for this coming week, because most fruits and vegetables become alkaline once they have been digested and broken down into other chemical components.

Vegan-Friendly Dietary Fats

There are a wide variety of ingredients vegans and vegetarians can include in their intermittent fasting regimes and still generate higher energy and fat stores.

If you have convictions or dietary restrictions that don't lend themselves to the high fat diets that meats tend to offer, here are five ways to add healthy high fat foods into your diet. And you don't have to be vegetarian or vegan to enjoy them.

1. Avocados

If you are a vegan, you should be stocking avocados in your fridge at all times. They lend themselves to any recipe that requires a creamy base. That very creaminess is a hint that they are high in fats – the healthy monounsaturated kind.

2. Coconut Oil

Unfortunately, clarified butter isn't an option for vegans because it is dairy. If you are vegan, try coconut oil instead. The flavor is fabulous, and it has a high smoking point which means you can deep fry almost anything in it. Coconut oil is a good source of medium-chain triglycerides which can be metabolized in the liver and used directly as an energy source.

3. Cocoa

When I talk about cocoa, I am not talking about hot chocolate and certainly not the candy that comes in wrappers. I am talking about the pure cocoa that comes in melted or powder form. Dark chocolate without the dairy and the sugar is a great source of energy and fat and should be part of your desert options.

4. Seeds

You can add seeds to all kinds of dishes or eat them on the side. They typically pack a large energy punch. Seeds are naturally designed to hold concentrated energy for the new plant until it can start extracting its own from the soil and sun.

One of the most nutritious seeds is the Inca Peanut. You can find them online by searching for "Savi Seed." They have loads of omega-3 and other nutrients. If you want to add them to soups and salads, they provide a good counter balance to spices and herbs. They are as much a super food as chia seeds and sunflower seeds. Consume them with meals during the induction and intermediate week if you can. They will help retrain your appetite for more places to find omega-3 and omega-6.

On the topic of omega-3 and omega-6, it is possible to have too much omega-3. In fact, there is a magic ratio for staying healthy. Ideally, you should have 1 portion of omega-3 to 4-6 parts of omega-6.

5. Nuts

Seeds and nuts are very different things. Seeds are the parts that grow into a new plant. Put them into the ground, water them, and they will sprout. Nuts, on the other hand, have hard shells that reveal the fruit inside when opened. A seed may be still further inside.

Nuts typically contain lots of protein and monounsaturated fats, and are great for vegans and vegetarians who aren't including meat fats and proteins in their diets. For non-vegetarians, nuts can introduce too many carbohydrates. Don't stop eating nuts, but simply be aware of it, and eat less if necessary.

21 Recipes

You can eat anything you want or your heart desires, as long as it is within a certain "window" of time, and it doesn't include processed foods.

Typical intermittent fasting diets don't say anything about the nutritional density of foods, or what you can and cannot eat, but if all you do is to fast intermittently, while continuing to poison your body with chemicals and processed foods, then not only is intermittent fasting going to be harder to do, it's also going to give you fewer results, and, eventually, you will give up.

So, let's just stick to eating healthy. Beyond that, you can eat as much as you feel like eating, and you can eat anything you like, just within specific widows of time while you get used to the process.

ABC Omelet (Apple, Bacon, Cheese)

2 tablespoons clarified butter, melted

3 slices streaky bacon

1 granny smith apple, cubed

2 eggs, whisked

2 oz. (57 g) blue cheese, crumbled

Melt the butter in a skillet and fry the bacon until crispy. Remove the bacon onto a paper towel. Add the cubed apple to the skillet and toss over medium heat. Reduce heat to low and continue cooking until the apple pieces turn golden. When they do, remove, and set aside.

Continue with the same skillet, using the remaining grease from the clarified butter and the bacon, increasing the heat to medium. Add the eggs and blue cheese and cook.

You shouldn't need to add salt — but if you do want to add more salt to taste, wait until the dish is served.

Serve the omelet on a plate, topped with the bacon and apples.

Yield: 1 serving

Aioli Fish

1 fillet white fish

2 tablespoons aioli (see recipe in induction week)

2 tablespoons parmesan cheese, grated

2 tablespoons clarified butter

Preheat oven to 340° F (170° C).

Spread aioli over both sides of the fish. Sprinkle both sides with parmesan.

Grease a baking pan with clarified butter. Place the fillet on the baking pan. Bake for 25 minutes furthest from the heat source.

Yield: 1 serving

Broiled Cod

6 cod fillets

¼ cup olive oil

3 tablespoons white wine vinegar

½ cup clarified butter, melted

1 tablespoon lemon juice

1 tablespoon spicy mustard

1 clove garlic, crushed

sea salt

ground black pepper

1 tablespoon fresh basil, chopped

Preheat the oven to 350° F (175° C).

Put the fish into a Ziplock bag. Add olive oil and vinegar and shake well.

Remove fish from bag and lay out in a baking pan lined with parchment. Bake until cooked through.

Combine clarified butter, lemon juice, mustard, garlic, salt, and pepper in a food processor. Run until smooth.

To serve, pour sauce over the fish, and sprinkle with basil.

Yield: 3 servings

By the Border Omelet

3 eggs

½ red onion, diced

habanero peppers, diced

2 tablespoons clarified butter

Monterey jack cheese, cubed

jalapeño jack cheese, cubed

tabasco sauce

sea salt

ground black pepper

3 tablespoons salsa

Whisk the eggs in a bowl until foamy. Drop in the diced peppers and onions.

Melt clarified butter in a skillet until it starts to sizzle. Tilt the skillet with one hand, allowing the sizzling butter to pool on one side of the tipped skillet. Use your free hand to pour the whisked eggs into the pool of butter. Level and return the skillet to the stove. This technique reduces the possibility of the eggs burning or cooking unevenly.

Sprinkle the cubed cheeses evenly over the eggs. Add salt, pepper, and a few dashes of tobasco sauce to taste.

Serve the cooked omelete warm topped with salsa.

Yield: 1 serving

Denver Omelet

2 tablespoons clarified butter

2 eggs

¼ small onion, sliced

1 oz. (28 g) cheddar cheese, shredded

¼ c. cooked ham, diced

¼ green pepper, sliced

sriracha chili sauce (optional)

Whisk the eggs and onions in a bowl until foamy.

Melt clarified butter in a small skillet until it starts to sizzle. Tilt the skillet with one hand and allow the sizzling butter to pool on one side. Using your free hand, pour the whisked eggs into the butter. Level the skillet and return it to the stove. This technique reduces the possibility of the eggs burning or cooking unevenly.

Sprinkle ham, cheese, and green pepper into the uncooked portion of the eggs. When partially cooked, flip it all over to finish cooking.

Add salt and pepper to taste.

This goes well with sriracha chili sauce if you want some added zing.

Yield: 1 serving

Ceviche

32 oz. (900 g) fresh fish (your choice), filleted

10 green limes (avg. size), juiced, seeds removed

3 green limes (avg. size), juiced separately, seeds removed

4 ripe tomatoes, skinned, seeds and core removed, diced

2 black avocados, skinned, cored, diced

3 fresh jalapeños, skinned, cored, finely diced

½ red onion, skinned, diced

1/3 cup fresh oregano, chopped

1/3 cup fresh cilantro, chopped

sea salt

ground black pepper

For this dish to work, everything must be fresh. Nothing can be frozen and thawed. Once a fish has been frozen and thawed, it affects the texture and taste of this dish.

Cut the fish fillet into bite-sized pieces and put into a crock or another similar container. Pour the juice of the 10 limes over the fish. Gently toss the fish and bath it in the juice until all the fish is fully coated.

(There should be enough lime juice that the fish floats freely in it.) Cover and marinate overnight in the fridge for a total of 12 hours. Toss the ingredients frequently before you turn in for the night, and then again when you wake in the morning. This step will cure the raw fish. The fish is "cooked" when all of it has turned white.

Combine tomatoes, jalapenos, avocado, and red onion in a separate bowl.

After marinating the fish, drain the lime juice. Gently remove the fish from the crock or container and add the drained fish to the bowl containing the diced vegetables.

Add cilantro, oregano, salt, and black pepper to the juice of the three remaining limes. Pour this juice mixture onto the fish and vegetables and toss. Serve chilled.

Yield: 3 servings for dinner (or 6 servings as an appetizer)

Cheesy Omelet

2 tablespoons clarified butter

2 eggs

2 oz. (57 g) cheddar cheese, shredded

2 oz. (57 g) monterey jack cheese, shredded

1 oz. (28 g) swiss cheese, chopped

fine sea salt

ground black pepper

lemon wedge

Use an electric whisk to aerate the eggs as you beat them - the more froth and foam, the better. Add a dash of salt to the eggs.

Melt the clarified butter in a small skillet over low heat until it starts to sizzle. Tilt the skillet with one hand and allow the sizzling butter to pool on one side. Use your free hand to pour the whisked eggs into that pool of butter. Level the skillet and return it to the stove. This reduces the possibility of the eggs burning or cooking unevenly.

As the bottom cooks sprinkle the shredded cheeses over the eggs.

Fold the omelet over and cook until a knife stuck in the middle comes out clean.

Slide the omelet out onto a plate to serve. Garnish with salt, pepper, and lemon.

Yield: 1 serving

Cheezy Lamb

½ lb. (228 g) roast lamb, cubed

sea salt

5-8 tbsp. clarified butter

1 onion, chopped

4 tablespoons parmesan cheese

3 tablespoons mayonnaise

2 eggs

Salt lamb and set aside to rest in a colander. The salt will pull out excess moisture from the meat.

Melt 2 tablespoons of the clarified butter in a skillet over medium heat until the butter sizzles. Sauté the lamb cubes till golden brown. Add the onion to the lamb and continue frying until softened. Set aside to cool.

Once cooled, add the lamb and onions to a food processor. Also add the parmesan cheese, mayonnaise, and any butter that remains in the skillet. Run the food processor until thoroughly mixed. Remove mixture from the food processor and set aside.

In a bowl, whisk the eggs and 3 tablespoons of the clarified butter together until foamy.

Melt 2 tablespoons of clarified butter in a skillet until it starts to sizzle. Tilt the skillet with one hand, allowing the melted butter to pool on one side. Use your free hand to pour the eggs into the pool of butter. Level the skillet and return it to the stove. This method reduces the possibility of the eggs burning or cooking unevenly.

Dump the lamb mix into the cooking eggs and fold twice.

Yield: 1 serving

Chinese Steamed Fish

12 oz. (340 g) cod fillet

2 teaspoons fresh ginger, grated

½ teaspoon fresh garlic, minced

1 tablespoon chinese rice wine

1 tablespoon soy sauce

1½ teaspoons toasted sesame oil

2 scallions, minced

You need a deep wok or skillet with a steamer rack that can support a shallow aluminum platter, and a lid to cover everything.

Bring water to a boil in the wok or skillet.

Lightly salt the cod, and sprinkle with grated ginger and garlic. Lay the cod out on the aluminum platter. Place the platter with the cod onto the steamer rack in the wok or skillet. Cover.

Mix rice wine, soy sauce, sesame oil, and scallions in a separate bowl.

Once the cod is fully steamed (the flesh will turn translucent white), remove it from the wok or skillet, and drizzle the soy sauce mixture over it. Serve immediately.

Yield: 2 servings

Cream Baked Sole

1 lb. (454 g) sole fillets

1 cup plain yogurt

½ cup mayonnaise

juice of 1 lemon

paprika

clarified butter

Preheat oven to 330°F (165° C).

Whisk together yogurt, mayonnaise, lemon juice, and paprika. Divide the mixture into two equal portions. One will be used to bake the fish; reserve the other to use as a dip.

Grease a baking dish with clarified butter. Lay soul fillets out in the dish. Spread one portion of the sauce mix over the fillets. Bake in oven for 40 minutes.

Once done, serve with reserved sauce on the side.

Yield: 3 servings

English Muffins

½ cup warm water

½ cup yogurt

1 teaspoon salt

2 ½ oz. (70 g) wheat gluten

¼ cup psyllium husk

2 tablespoons wheat germ

¼ cup wheat bran

½ cup oat flour

½ cup whey powder

2 drops vanilla extract

2 teaspoons yeast

2 tablespoons clarified butter

Combine all ingredients except the clarified butter in a mixer with a dough hook attachment. Once mixed, use a damp cloth to cover the bowl with the dough, and set aside for 30 minutes.

Return bowl to the mixer and run on low setting for 30 seconds. Remove dough and lay out on a clean surface. Flatten and spread the dough out into a ½ in. (1.25 cm) thick square. Using a circular dough cutter, cut out 2-4 circles. Gather the excess dough into a ball, flatten, and cut out more circles. Lay dough circles out on a greased pan, cover with a clean damp cloth, and allow to rise.

Melt clarified butter in a heavy skillet over low heat, thoroughly coating the skillet. Place the risen dough circles neatly into the skillet and cover. Fry until the sides turn brown, then flip them over. Continue cooking until you are confident they are completely cooked through on the inside.

Yield: About 6-7 muffins

Ginger Salmon

1 salmon fillet, skin on

1 clove fresh garlic, crushed

½ inch fresh ginger root, grated

2 tablespoons fresh cilantro, chopped

2 scallions, minced

½ cup white wine

2 tablespoons clarified butter

sea salt

ground black pepper

8 tablespoons sour cream

Combine garlic, ginger, cilantro, scallions, and white wine.

Heat the clarified butter in a heavy skillet and sauté the salmon for 4 minutes on each side. Add the white wine/herb mixture to the skillet. Cook for another 3 minutes. Season to taste with salt and pepper.

To serve, spoon the sauce over the fish, and top with a generous dollop of sour cream.

Yield: 2 servings

Homemade Sour Cream

6 tablespoons buttermilk

2 cups heavy cream

Make the sour cream 2 days ahead of use.

Mix the heavy cream with the buttermilk. Leave in the bottom shelf of the fridge for two days.

Flounder Tarragon & Asparagus

26 oz. (750 g) flounder fillet

30 asparagus spears

sea salt

homemade sour cream (as above)

juice of 1 lemon

Prepare asparagus by snapping woody part off each spear at the base. Bring a pot of salted water to a boil. Drop in the asparagus. Cook for 3 minutes, remove, and blanch in cold running water.

In a separate bowl, mix the homemade sour cream, mustard, and tarragon.

Sprinkle the flounder with sea salt and coat with aioli. Heat a skillet and add two tablespoons of clarified butter and sauté the fish fillet. Once cooked, remove the flounder, leaving excess oil in the skillet.

Place the fish on a serving plate. Drizzle with lemon juice. Place a dollop of the sour cream sauce on the fish. Carefully lay out asparagus on that.

Yield: 2 servings

Pan-Seared Sea Bass

2 lbs. (907 g) sea bass fillets

juice of 1 lemon

2 tablespoon Old Bay Seasoning

8 slices bacon

½ cup clarified butter, melted

Slice the fillets into serving-sized pieces. Gently toss to thoroughly coat the fish in half of the lemon juice. Sprinkle the fish evenly with Old Bay Seasoning.

Use a deep skillet and render the bacon. Remove the bacon, leaving the bacon fat. Fry the sea bass in the sizzling bacon grease for 4 minutes. Flip, and fry for another 4 minutes.

To serve, pour clarified butter over the fish, and sprinkle with remaining lemon juice. Garnish with bacon pieces.

Yield: 6 servings

Pork Frittatas

12 eggs

½ cup parmesan cheese, grated

1 tablespoon lard

½ lb. (225 g) pork sausage, crumbled

½ cup sweet red onion, diced

½ cup green pepper, diced

½ cup sweet red pepper, diced

1 teaspoon fine sea salt

You will need a skillet that can go in the oven and an oven with a broiler.

Beat the eggs in a bowl for 3-4 minutes. Add the parmesan cheese.

Melt the lard in the skillet over medium heat. Add crumbled sausage and brown. When the sausage is light brown, add the onions and continue stirring until the onions soften. Then add green peppers. Sprinkle lightly with salt. Distribute the meat and vegetables evenly in the bottom of the pan. Reduce to low heat.

Pour the beaten eggs over the contents of the skillet. Cover the skillet with an oven-safe lid or aluminum foil and cook for 2 minutes.

Move the covered skillet into the oven, under the broiler, and cook for 10 minutes.

Yield: 6 servings

Rice Bran Bread

9 ½ oz. (270 ml) water

1 oz. (30 g) rice bran

3/4 oz. (20 g) flaxseed meal

3 ½ oz. (100 g) wheat gluten

1 ½ oz. (40 g) whey protein powder

2 teaspoons blackstrap molasses

1 teaspoon sea salt

½ oz. (15 ml) clarified butter

2 teaspoons yeast

A bread maker is required.

Put all ingredients into the bread maker. Set the program for light or dark skin, as desired.

Yield: 10 slices

Sautéed Sole in Balsamic Vinegar

2 lbs. (907 g) sole fillets

white wine vinegar

sea salt

ground black pepper

4 tablespoons clarified butter

½ cup white wine

1 tablespoon fresh oregano

¼ cup balsamic vinegar

2 tablespoon olive oil

1 cup shredded Parmesan cheese

3 lemon wedges

Place the sole fillets in a bowl. Pour in the white wine vinegar and sloshing it around to rinse all the fish. Once the fish has been rinsed in it, discard the vinegar, and lay the fish out on paper towels to dry.

Sprinkle the fish with salt and pepper. Gently rub the seasoning into both sides of the fish with your hands.

Melt butter in a skillet and heat until sizzling. Sauté the fillets on both sides. Use a slotted spoon and a wooden spatula to hold the fillets carefully as you turn them over.

Pour the white wine into the skillet, without pouring it on the fish. Let the wine slowly sizzle, allowing the alcohol to evaporate. Sprinkle the oregano over the fish. Continue cooking until the wine fully evaporates.

Remove the sole from the skillet and lay out on a plate. Add the balsamic vinegar, drizzle with olive oil, and sprinkle with parmesan cheese. Serve with a wedge of lemon on the side.

Yield: 3 servings

Sea Bass in Heavy Cream

12 oz. (340 g) sea bass filleted

3 tablespoons olive oil

½ lb. (225 g) mixed olives, pitted, washed

2 anchovy fillets, sliced

2 tablespoons capers

2 fresh basil leaves, crushed

juice of 1 lemon

2 tablespoons extra virgin olive oil

2 tablespoons clarified butter

¼ onion, sliced thinly

2 cloves garlic, crushed

1 tablespoon balsamic vinegar

3 tablespoons heavy cream

sea salt

ground black pepper

Pre-heat broiler. Divide sea bass fillets into two portions. Brush 3 tablespoons of olive oil on all sides. Broil the fish as you prepare the sauce.

To make tapenade, combine the olives, anchovies, capers, basil, lemon juice, and the 2 tablespoons extra virgin olive oil in a food processor. Run until you get a smooth paste. Set aside.

Sauté onions and garlic with the 2 tablespoons of butter in a heavy skillet for 5 minutes. Add the tapenade and balsamic vinegar to the skillet. Continue sautéing for 2 minutes. Remove from heat and let rest for 2 minutes. Stir in the cream.

Spoon the sauce over the fish to serve. Add salt and pepper to taste.

Yield: 2 servings

Spanish Tilapia

4 whole tilapias filleted

¾ teaspoon paprika

juice of 3 limes

2 tablespoons clarified butter

½ cup clarified butter

1 medium red onion, thinly sliced

¼ teaspoon ground cumin

3 tablespoons orange juice

½ teaspoon habanero sauce

1 tablespoon white wine vinegar

1 tablespoon fresh oregano

sea salt

ground black pepper

Arrange the tilapia fillets on a flat plate. Mix 1/3 of the lime juice in a separate bowl with the paprika. Drench both sides of the fish with the juice mixture.

Melt 2 tablespoons butter in a heavy skillet and sauté fillets until golden on each side. Remove fish and place in an oven-safe serving dish. Keep dish warm in the oven. Leave the grease in the skillet.

Add the ½ cup of clarified butter to the skillet, melting it over medium heat. When it sizzles, add the onions, and sauté until soft and brown. Add cumin, stirring until fragrant. Add remaining lime juice, orange juice, habanero sauce, white wine vinegar, and oregano. Stir over medium-low heat for about 2 minutes.

To serve, spoon the onion sauce over the tilapia.

Yield: 4 servings

Tilapia with Vegetables

1 lb. (454 g) tilapia fillets

sea salt

white pepper

3 tablespoons clarified butter

2 cups red pepper, sliced

2 cups yellow pepper, sliced

2 cups zucchini, sliced

2 cups squash, diced

2 cups red onion, diced

1 clove garlic, crushed

¾ tablespoon corn flour

lemon wedges

Rub the sea salt and white pepper onto the tilapia fillets and set aside.

Melt the butter in a skillet. Sauté the vegetables, onions, and garlic for 4 to 5 minutes, stirring frequently. Lay the fish over the vegetables in the skillet, and cover. Keep heat at medium. Cook for 10 minutes in the steam.

Lay out the fish out on a serving dish and shimmy the vegetables onto the fish, retaining the liquids in the skillet. Return the skillet to the heat, and when the sauce is sizzling, add in the corn flour, continuing to stir until the sauce thickens. Pour the thickened sauce over the vegetables and fish. Serve with lemon wedges.

Yield: 4 servings

Chapter 5: Advanced "Booster" Week

Advanced "Booster" Week is all about boosting the way your body asks for food. By getting your metabolism to switch tracks for longer periods of time, you can be a continuous fat-burning machine rather than a fat-storing machine.

"Booster" Schedule

This schedule is fairly easy to follow. It is organized according to "windows" of time. During 2-hour meal windows, you have full meals — full meals are defined as whatever you want to eat and however much you can eat without feeling over-full. The key is to always listen to your body. These are alternated with fasting no-meal windows. During those periods of fasting, remember to keep drinking the lemon water, and stay hydrated.

			DAY				
Meal	1	2	3	4	5	6	7
7am -9am	0	MD2	0	0	MD5	0	0
11am - 1pm	0	0	0	0	0	0	0
6pm - 8pm	ED1	0	0	ED4	0	0	ED7

The basic schedule follows a 7:2 pattern. Two meal windows follow each other, ED1 and MD2, for instance. These are followed by seven windows of no meals. That is followed by two meal time windows and another seven fasting windows. This 7:2 formula is designed to alter the metabolism, activating the body's fat-burning metabolism for longer periods. The foods in the booster week recipes below will also help with that goal.

10 Recipes

Chicken Pie

2 lbs. (907 g) chicken (dark, no skin), chopped

1 quart (1.1 L) chicken broth

2 tablespoons clarified butter

1 cup baking flour

¼ lb. (115 g) carrots, diced

¼ lb. (115 g) peas

¼ lb. (115 g) green beans, cut in ½ inch pieces

1 cup shitake mushrooms, sliced

1 cup almond milk

sea salt

ground black pepper

corn flour

Put chopped chicken and broth into a pressure cooker. Pressurize and cook for 30 minutes.

Once the chicken is done, release the pressure and open the cover. Remove the chicken pieces and drain in a colander. Remove and strain one cup of broth, leaving the remaining broth in the pot.

Combine the strained cup of broth, baking flour, and clarified butter in a mixing bowl. Knead until it forms a soft dough, then fold it over on itself numerous times.

Flour a flat surface and lay the dough on it. Use a rolling pin to flatten the dough. Fold it again, then roll it. Repeat five times. The dough should be ¼ inch thick.

Line the inside of an oven-safe glass bowl with the flattened dough, letting the excess hang over the sides. Set aside.

Add the vegetables (carrots, peas, green beans, and mushrooms) to the hot broth in the pot. Cook for about 4-5 minutes. Add the almond milk. Add corn flour to the broth and keep stirring until it thickens. Season with salt and pepper.

Return the chicken to the pot with the thickened broth and veggies. Mix thoroughly.

Scoop the chicken, vegetables, and gravy into the dough-lined bowl. Fold the excess dough back on top of it.

Bake in the oven for 20 minutes.

Serve warm, using a large serving spoon to scoop out the crust and chicken mixture.

Yield: 6 servings

Dumplings

1 quart (1.1 L) chicken broth

1 cup ground almonds

½ cup rice protein powder

¼ cup wheat flour

2 tablespoons clarified butter

2 tablespoons coconut oil

½ teaspoon fine sea salt

2 teaspoons baking powder

½ teaspoon baking soda

¾ cup plain yogurt

Set the chicken broth to boil in a pot.

Pulse all remaining ingredients, except the yogurt, in a food processor until fully mixed. Add the yogurt and fold everything together. You should now have a soft dough.

Using a spoon, scoop half-tablespoons of the dough and drop into the boiling broth. Cook over medium-high heat for 30 minutes.

Yield: 12 servings

Egg Drop Soup

1 quart (1.1 L) chicken broth

1 tablespoon coconut aminos (soy sauce replacement)

1 tablespoon umeboshi vinegar (ume plum vinegar)

½ teaspoon fresh ginger, grated

1 scallion, finely sliced

2 eggs

ground white pepper

Heat the broth in a saucepan over medium-high heat. Add coconut amino, umeboshi vinegar, ginger, and scallion. Simmer for 4 minutes.

Beat the eggs lightly in a bowl.

Once the broth is boiling, pour the beaten egg into the broth, slowly as one continuous stream . Don't pour the egg all at once or drip it in. Pour the egg in one long, controlled stream, while stirring the broth in a circular motion.

Serve with pepper to taste.

Yield: 4 Servings

Ground Beef Stir-Fry

1 lb. (454 g) ground beef

2 tablespoons coconut aminos

3 tablespoons chinese cooking wine

2 cloves garlic, crushed

sea salt

3 tablespoons (or more) coconut oil

½ cup peanuts, coarsely chopped

1½ teaspoons fresh ginger, grated

1 cup green beans, chopped

1 cup broccoli, chopped

1 medium onion, sliced

1 teaspoon fish sauce

Combine 1 tablespoon of the coconut aminos, 1 tablespoon of the cooking wine, a pinch of sea salt and the garlic. Massage that into the ground beef. Separate the ground beef mix into bite-sized chunks.

Heat 3 tablespoons coconut oil in a deep wok over high heat. Fry the peanuts until golden. Remove and set aside.

Fry the ground beef chunks in the oil after removing the peanuts. Remove the beef.

Add more oil if necessary and sauté the ginger until fragrant. Remove and set aside.

Fry the green beans, broccoli, and onion for 2-4 minutes until cooked. Return the beef, peanuts, and ginger to the wok. Toss everything together, adding the fish sauce, remaining coconut aminos, and remaining cooking wine.

Yield: 3 servings

Lemon-Glazed Turkey Cutlets

3 turkey breasts, cubed

rosemary, finely chopped

1 tablespoon clarified butter

1 tablespoon lemon juice

½ teaspoon coconut aminos

3 scallions, thinly sliced

sea salt

ground black pepper

Pulse turkey, rosemary, and salt in a food processor until the meat is chunky. Form the mixture into patties by hand.

Heat clarified butter in a heavy skillet until sizzling. Fry the turkey patties until brown. Remove and set aside.

Combine lemon juice, coconut aminos, scallions, salt, and pepper. Heat this lemon juice mixture in the skillet. Pour this glaze over the turkey patties before serving.

Yield: 2 or 3 servings

Mushroom Turkey Wings

4 lbs. (1.8 Kg) turkey wings

1 cup clarified butter

½ medium onion, sliced

1 cup mushrooms, sliced

1 tablespoon tomato paste

½ cup chicken broth

sea salt

1 tablespoon corn flour

½ cup sour cream

Melt butter in a cast iron dutch oven over high heat until sizzling. Pan fry the turkey wings until brown. Add onions and fry until brown. Add the mushrooms. Cover and cook for 10 minutes.

Stir in the tomato paste. Add the chicken broth. Season with sea salt. Cover and boil for 10 minutes.

Remove turkey wings and set aside.

Stir corn flour into the pan to thicken the broth. Add sour cream and stir.

Serve the turkey wings with the sauce.

Yield: 3 servings

Mustard Turkey Cutlets

3 turkey breast cutlets or turkey breasts

½ cup raw almonds

1 tablespoon chinese hot mustard

3 tablespoons eggless mayonnaise

3 tablespoons clarified butter

Brown almonds in a dry frypan. Use a food processor to chop the almonds until fine. Add the mustard and eggless mayonnaise and continue blending.

Coat the turkey with the almond mix.

Melt butter in a heavy skillet until sizzling. Fry turkey until browned.

To serve, pour the grease from the pan and any almond scrapings over the turkey.

Yield: 2 Servings

Prosciutto Salad

14 oz. (400 g) artichoke hearts, cut in bite-sized pieces

3.5 oz. (100 g) prosciutto, thinly sliced, cut into 1 x ¼ inch pieces (25 x 6 mm)

½ cup pitted olives, chopped

1 large tomato, skinned and diced

¼ cup fresh basil, finely chopped

3 tablespoons extra virgin olive oil

4 teaspoons white wine vinegar

2 cloves garlic, crushed

½ teaspoon spicy mustard

Combine artichoke hearts, prosciutto strips, olive pieces, diced tomato, and basil in a bowl. Toss together.

Combine olive oil, vinegar, garlic, and mustard. Add this dressing to the bowl and toss all together thoroughly.

Let sit for 20 minutes in the fridge before serving.

Yield: 4 servings

Stracciatella

1 tablespoon bacon grease

1 fresh rosemary sprig, finely chopped

½ teaspoon fresh nutmeg, grated

1 quart (1.1 L) chicken broth

2 eggs, lightly beaten

1 tablespoon balsamic vinegar

1 tablespoon lemon juice

ground black pepper to taste

½ cup grated parmesan cheese

Heat bacon grease in pot. Sauté rosemary and nutmeg. Add chicken broth and bring to boil. Pour beaten eggs into the boiling soup while stirring. When the eggs are firm, add vinegar, lemon juice, and pepper.

Distribute broth to serving sized oven-safe bowls. Top with parmesan cheese. Place under broiler until the cheese melts. Serve warm.

Yield: 4 servings

Submarine Salad

8 cups rocket lettuce

½ lb. (227 g) prosciutto

¼ lb. (113 g) mortadella

¼ lb. (113 g) salami

¼ lb. (113 g) smoked provolone cheese, sliced

¼ lb. (113 g) mozzarella cheese, sliced

1 red onion, sliced

3 tablespoons roasted red pepper, chopped

4 fresh basil leaves, chopped

1 large tomato, skinned, cored and sliced

2 tablespoons extra virgin olive oil

1 clove garlic, crushed

1 tablespoon red wine vinegar

pinch ground black pepper

pinch sea salt

Make a bed of rocket lettuce on a large serving plate.

Slice all the cheese and meats into strips 1 inch (2.5 cm) long by ¼ inch (.6 cm) wide.

On the bed of lettuce, layer a little cheese, then a little meat, then a little cheese again, alternating the sliced ingredients.

Just before serving, top with the onions, red pepper, basil, and tomato.

Blend olive oil, garlic, wine vinegar, black pepper, and salt to make a dressing. Pour this dressing over all the ingredients on the serving platter.

Yield: 2 servings

A Healthy Intermittent Fasting Lifestyle

Having reached the end of three weeks of intermittent fasting, you are now truly a new person, functioning in a different way, restoring your mind and body to a way of consuming food that is more in line with that of our ancestors of 50,000 years ago. These three weeks of discipline have been designed to change the body in such a way that it has stopped responding to food in habitual ways and has therefore stopped being derailed by those habits. The idea has been to get your body to make the right choices regardless of what the mind is saying.

During the past three weeks, you have also been scrubbed of the toxins usually contained in processed foods, allowing you to be truer to your natural appetites. You won't just crave flavorful or pleasing foods that have empty calories but you will have an appetite for the things your body really needs.

Shifting how your body asks for food is an important element in eating healthy, but we went one step further. Not only did we start getting your body to ask for the right food, we got your body to ask for it at the right time, when it needed it. We changed the basic philosophy of eating: now we look to stored food to energize us instead of eating to increase stores.

We also looked to expand the range of food choices, rather than restricting it. Fasts that cut out what you eat and reduce it to certain areas are not healthy because they reduce the diversity of your choices. Our body needs hundreds of different compounds (enzymes, vitamins, minerals, proteins, and more), so we cannot just limit our diet to a few food sources. The more you diversify your foods, the more your body will get what it needs, and will add to its "library" of sources for what it needs.

The "what" and "when" of eating is what intermittent fasting is all about. The "when" is easy to discern – we eat when our body needs it. The "what" is anything we want to eat – as long as it isn't processed or something that harms us.

Now, having gotten this far, you should stop looking at the eating schedules as rigid plans and begin to see them as guardrails. That means you should eat what you feel like and only when you feel hungry. If you find you are eating too often and/or too much, and the weight is creeping back on, then you can pull back. Otherwise, leave the timing of meals, the amount to eat, and the items to eat to the dictates of your own body. Remember, weight loss can occur naturally in intermittent fasting because stored fat is being used as fuel.

Not only do you have access to a higher quality source of energy when you do this, you also allow the body more time to clean up, get healthy, and get alert. Remember when we talked about the protein shells – those "bags" that carry fats to their destinations? The body needs time to clean that up. Fasting perfectly provides time for your body to digest and flush all those protein packets out of your system after they have been used. That is the reason my LDL levels dropped after my first 30-day fast. Intermittent fasting gives your body time to make repairs to all its issues.

I especially want to remind you to drink plenty of water. You don't have to add lemon to your water anymore if you don't want to. The lemon was added mostly to shift your intake toward the alkaline side of the equation because most processed foods are notorious acidifying foods. Switching to a more alkaline diet should have helped to readjust your taste buds.

You should also continue to stay away from sugar – and that really does include sugar substitutes like stevia and all those aspartame derivatives. It is not so much that they are bad for you as that they encourage the habit of wanting sweetness. Learn to take foods as they are without adding the taste of sweet. That sweetness is the lazy way out in terms of energy generation. Sugars give you a quick boost of energy but are never enough to keep you going for long. Triglycerides are a better source of energy and you can get that everywhere because your body makes them from almost everything you eat. Eating healthy foods starts by skewing your taste preferences and cravings toward what is healthy.

Final Thoughts

This brings us to the end of this book on intermittent fasting. I hope it has been of help to you and that you have found the inspiration to experience a new way of eating that will elevate your body's ability to meet its full potential. Intermittent fasting will change the way you move, the way you think, and the way you succeed in all the things that you do.

Happy living!

If you enjoyed learning about Intermittent Fasting I would be forever grateful if you could leave a review on Amazon. Reviews are by far the best way to help your fellow readers find the good books so make sure to help them out!

Appendix: List of Acidic Foods PH

The following is a list of foods with their corresponding pH values. Acidic foods have a pH between 1 and 6.9 – the lower the number the more acidic. Neutral is a pH of 7. Alkaline is from 7.1 to 14. The higher the number, the higher the alkalinity.

Most of the items in this list are fruits and vegetables. Most fruits and vegetables become alkaline in the body after they have been digested, even though they start out as acidic.

Item	Approximate pH
Lemons / Lemon Juice	2.0
Limes / Lime Juice	2.0
Cranberry Juice, canned	2.3
Grenadine Syrup	2.3
Vinegar	2.4
Gelatin Dessert	2.6
Loganberries	2.7
Chili Sauce, acidified	2.8
Gooseberries	2.8
Grapes, Concord	2.8

Grapes, Niagara	2.8
Plums, Blue	2.8
Raspberry Jam	2.9
Grapes, Seedless	2.9
Grapefruit Juice, canned	2.9
Plums, Damson	2.9
Crabapple Jelly	2.9
Pomegranate	2.9
Grapefruit	3.0
Fruit Jellies	3.0
Orange Marmalade	3.0
Strawberries	3.0
Strawberry Jam	3.0
Tamarind	3.0
Youngberries, frozen	3.0
Mint Jelly	3.0
Grapefruit, canned	3.1
Applesauce	3.1
Red Pepper Relish	3.1
Rhubarb	3.1
Cider Vinegar	3.1

Blueberries	3.1
Quince, fresh, stewed	3.1
Raspberries, fresh or frozen	3.2
Apple, baked with sugar	3.2
Cucumbers / Dill Pickles	3.2
Grapes, Muscatine	3.2
Pineapple	3.2
Rhubarb, California, stewed	3.2
Strawberries, frozen	3.2
Plums, frozen	3.2
Plums, Green Gage, canned	3.2
Cherries, red, water packed	3.3
Mayhaw	3.3
Peaches, frozen	3.3
Apricots	3.3
Apricots, dried, stewed	3.3
Orange Juice, California	3.3
Orange Juice, Florida	3.3
Peaches	3.3
Pineapple Juice, canned	3.3
Sauerkraut	3.3

Cherries, frozen	3.3
Strawberries, California	3.3
Tangerine	3.3
Apples, Jonathan	3.3
Apples, McIntosh	3.3
Apple Juice	3.4
Pineapple, canned	3.4
Guava, canned	3.4
Sherry Wine	3.4
Huckleberries, cooked with sugar	3.4
Apricots, canned	3.4
Mangoes, ripe	3.4
Rhubarb, canned	3.4
Apricots, pureed	3.4
Plum Nectar	3.5
Apples, Winesap	3.5
Cherries, Maraschino	3.5
Bamboo Shoots, preserved	3.5
Grapes, canned	3.5
Grapes, Tokyo	3.5
Fruit Jam	3.5

Pears, Bartlett	3.5
Raspberries, New Jersey	3.5
Tomatoes, canned	3.5
Tomato Paste	3.5
Grapes, Lady Finger	3.5
Papaya Marmalade	3.5
Mustard	3.6
Peaches, cooked with sugar	3.6
Apples, Golden Delicious	3.6
Fruit Cocktail	3.6
Olives, green, fermented	3.6
Oranges, Florida, "color added"	3.6
Plums, Green Gage	3.6
Plums, Red	3.6
Prunes, pureed	3.6
Prunes, dried, stewed	3.6
Worcestershire Sauce	3.6
Kumquat, Florida	3.6
Oranges, Florida	3.7
Raspberry Sherbet	3.7
Grapes, Ribier	3.7

Honey	3.7
Onions, pickled	3.7
Peaches, canned	3.7
Quince Jelly	3.7
Grapes, Malaga	3.7
Apricots, strained	3.7
Guava Jelly	3.7
Apricot Nectar	3.8
Cherries, Royal Ann	3.8
Coconut Preserves	3.8
Raisins, seedless	3.8
Cherries, Black, canned	3.8
Tomatillos	3.8
Blackberries, Washington	3.9
Ketchup	3.9
Apples, Delicious	3.9
Plums, Yellow	3.9
Vegetable Juice	3.9
Nectarines	3.9
Prune Juice	4.0
Pears, canned	4.0

Cherries, California	4.0
Pear Nectar	4.0
Pears, Sickle, cooked w/sugar	4.0
Acidophilus Milk	4.1
Cream Cheese, Philadelphia	4.1
Tomato Juice	4.1
Dates, Dromedary	4.1
Cucumbers, pickled	4.2
Artichokes, canned, acidified	4.3
Beets, canned, acidified	4.3
Tomatoes	4.3
Enchilada sauce	4.4
Pimiento/Pimento	4.4
Soy Sauce	4.4
Buttermilk	4.4
Persimmons	4.4
Tomatoes, vine ripened	4.4
Bananas	4.5
Pickled Herring	4.5
Mangosteen	4.5
Taro syrup	4.5

Carrots, pureed	4.6
Bananas, red	4.6
Curry Paste, acidified	4.6
Maple Syrup, light (acidified)	4.6
Cream of Tomato Soup, canned	4.6
Peppers	4.7
Cactus	4.7
Honey Aloe	4.7
Lychee	4.7
Sour Milk, fine curd	4.7
Cottage Cheese	4.8
Asparagus	4.8
Jackfruit	4.8
Zwiebach	4.8
Basil Pesto	4.9
Beets, canned	4.9
Corn Flakes	4.9
Molasses	4.9
Peas, pureed	4.9
Pumpkin	4.9
Rambutan (Thailand)	4.9

Straw Mushroom	4.9
Figs, canned	4.9
Fish Sauce	4.9
Cheese, American, mild	5.0
Vegetable Soup	5.0
Wheat Krispies	5.0
Abalone Mushrooms	5.0
Asparagus, canned	5.0
Banana, yellow	5.0
White Bread	5.0
Nata De Coco	5.0
Oyster Mushrooms	5.0
Satay Sauce	5.0
Shrimp Paste	5.0
Wheaties	5.0
Boston Style Beans	5.1
Figs, Calamyrna	5.1
Mixed Greens, chopped	5.1
Melba Toast	5.1
Bamboo Shoots	5.1

Pork & Beans with Tomato Sauce, canned	5.1
Carrots, strained	5.1
Cheese, Roquefort	5.1
Loquat (may be acidified to pH 3.8)	5.1
Macaroni, cooked	5.1
Potatoes, mashed	5.1
Cucumbers	5.1
Maple syrup	5.2
Vegetable Soup, canned	5.2
Carrots, canned	5.2
Cheese, Snippy	5.2
Acorn Squash, cooked	5.2
Watermelon	5.2
Barley, cooked	5.2
Asparagus, green, canned	5.2
Baby Corn	5.2
Rye Bread	5.2
Broccoli, canned	5.2
Cabbage	5.2
Cheese, Parmesan	5.2

Chives	5.2
Jujube	5.2
Papaya	5.2
Green Peppers	5.2
Rattan, Thailand	5.2
Mixed Greens, strained	5.2
Beets, cooked	5.2
Puffed Wheat	5.3
Turnips	5.3
Wax Beans	5.3
Beets	5.3
Carrots, chopped	5.3
Codfish, boiled	5.3
Milkfish	5.3
Parsnip	5.3
Shallots, cooked	5.3
Sweet Potatoes	5.3
Truffle	5.3
Beans with Tomato Sauce, canned	5.32
Beets, chopped or strained	5.3
Onions, yellow or red	5.3

Wheat Chex	5.3
Breadfruit, cooked	5.3
Horseradish, freshly ground	5.4
Salmon, fresh, broiled	5.4
Celery, cooked	5.4
Onions, white	5.4
Spinach, chopped	5.4
Kidney Beans	5.4
Pumpernickel Bread	5.4
Cheese, Edam	5.4
Potatoes	5.4
Rice Krispies	5.4
Three Bean Salad	5.4
Turnip Greens, cooked	5.4
Sardine, Portuguese, in olive oil	5.4
Walnuts, English	5.4
Cracked Wheat Bread	5.4
Bran Flakes	5.5
Parsnips, cooked	5.5
White Bread Rolls	5.5
Whole Wheat Bread	5.5

Fennel (Anise)	5.5
Leeks, cooked	5.5
Ackees	5.5
Artichokes	5.5
Cabbage, Green	5.5
Coconut, fresh	5.5
Eggplant	5.5
Guava Nectar	5.5
Leeks	5.5
Okra, cooked	5.5
Red Ginseng	5.5
Enchilada Sauce	5.5
Spinach	5.5
Spinach, pureed	5.5
Yams, cooked	5.5
Cream of Coconut, canned	5.5
Radishes, white	5.5
Squash, white, cooked	5.5
Turnip, yellow, cooked	5.6
Carrots, cooked	5.6
Antipasto	5.6

Artichokes, French, cooked	5.6
Beans	5.6
Beans, String	5.6
Cabbage, Red	5.6
Cauliflower	5.6
Four Bean Salad	5.6
Ginger	5.6
Spinach, strained	5.6
Soda Crackers	5.7
Yeast	5.7
Cheese, Swiss Gruyere	5.7
Oysters	5.7
Zucchini, cooked	5.7
Caviar, American	5.7
Celery	5.7
Cheese, Stilton	5.7
Escarole	5.7
Hearts of Palm	5.7
Lettuce, Iceberg	5.7
Lobster Soup	5.7
Matzos	5.7

Parsley	5.7
Peas, canned	5.7
Cream of Pea Soup, canned	5.7
Pork & Beans	5.7
Sardines	5.7
Shad Roe, sauteed	5.7
Celery Knob, cooked	5.7
Kippered Herring, Marshall	5.8
Turnip, white, cooked	5.8
Beans, Black	5.8
Melon, Casaba	5.8
Romaine Lettuce	5.8
Squash, yellow, cooked	5.8
Calamari (Squid)	5.8
Cheese Dip	5.8
Fennel, cooked	5.8
Garlic	5.8
Grass Jelly	5.8
Lentil Soup	5.8
Lettuce	5.8
Mangoes, green	5.8

Vermicelli, cooked	5.8
Radishes, red	5.9
Salmon, fresh, boiled	5.9
Wheatena	5.9
Carrots	5.9
Watercress	5.9
Lettuce, Boston	5.9
Beans, refried	5.9
Cheese, Cheddar	5.9
Chicory	5.9
Corn	5.9
Corn, canned	5.9
Mackerel, canned	5.9
Melons, Persian	5.9
Milk, evaporated	5.9
Pate	5.9
Potato Soup	5.9
Tuna Fish, canned	5.9
Peas, strained	5.9
Scotch Broth	5.9
Artichokes, Jerusalem, cooked	5.9

Baby Food Soup, unstrained	6.0
Cream of Mushroom Soup, canned	5.95
Spaghetti, cooked	6.0
Aloe Juice	6.0
Asparagus	6.0
Soybeans	6.0
Brussels Sprouts	6.0
Capers	6.0
Carp	6.0
Chayote (Mirliton), cooked	6.0
Clams	6.0
Cream of Potato Soup	6.0
Curry sauce	6.0
Korean Ginseng Drink	6.0
Hominy, cooked	6.0
Melons, Honeydew	6.0
Mushrooms	6.0
Mussels	6.0
Octopus	6.0
Olives, black	6.0

Olives, ripe	6.0
Oysters, smoked	6.0
Razor shell (sea asparagus)	6.0
Rice, White, cooked	6.0
Rice, Wild, cooked	6.0
Scallop	6.0
Sea Snail (Top shell)	6.0
Squash, Hubbard, cooked	6.0
Squid	6.0
Water Chestnut	6.0
Asparagus, cooked	6.0
Shredded Wheat	6.1
Cream of Wheat, cooked	6.1
Mackerel, Spanish, broiled	6.1
Salmon, Red Alaska, canned	6.1
Gelatin, plain	6.1
Noodles, boiled	6.1
Bluefish, Boston, broiled	6.1
Abalone	6.1
Aloe Vera	6.1
Asparagus Stalks	6.1

Coconut milk	6.1
Cream of Asparagus	6.1
Egg Yolk	6.1
Flounder, boiled	6.1
Herring	6.1
Cantaloupe	6.1
Cheese, Old English	6.2
Haddock, Filet, broiled	6.2
Swiss Chard, cooked	6.2
Cabbage, White	6.2
Cod Liver	6.2
Dates, canned	6.2
Eel	6.2
Oatmeal, cooked	6.2
Razor Clams	6.2
Rice, Brown, cooked	6.2
Scallion	6.2
Sturgeon	6.2
Trout, Sea, sautéed	6.2
Corn, cooked on cob	6.2
Peas, cooked	6.2

Mackerel, King, boiled	6.3
Avocados	6.3
Puffed Rice	6.3
Peanut Butter	6.3
Broccoli, cooked	6.3
Broccoli, frozen, cooked	6.3
Cabbage, Savoy	6.3
Cuttlefish	6.3
Kelp	6.3
Lentils, cooked	6.3
Spinach, frozen, cooked	6.3
Milk, condensed	6.3
Asparagus, frozen, cooked	6.4
Kale, cooked	6.4
Arrowroot Cruel	6.4
Flounder, fillet, broiled	6.4
Clam Chowder, New England	6.4
Congee	6.4
Milk, cow	6.4
Peas, frozen, cooked	6.4
Porgy, broiled	6.4

Peas, dried (split yellow), cooked	6.43
Cereal, strained	6.4
Cream, 40 per cent	6.4
Cauliflower, cooked	6.5
Peas, dried (split green), cooked	6.45
Milk, goat	6.5
Chick Peas / Garbanzo Beans	6.5
Anchovies	6.5
Striped Bass, broiled	6.5
Beans, Lima	6.5
Crab Meat	6.5
Cream, 20%	6.5
Chrysanthemum Drink	6.5
Shrimp	6.5
Bread, Boston, brown	6.5
Sea Bass, broiled	6.6
Eggs, new-laid, whole	6.6
Soy Infant Formula	6.6
Spinach, cooked	6.6
Crabmeat, cooked	6.6
Arrowroot Crackers	6.6

Smelts, sautéed	6.7
Asparagus Buds	6.7
Hearts of Palm	6.7
Pollack, fillet, broiled	6.7
Lobster Bisque	6.9
Lotus Root	6.9
Soybean Milk	7.0
Shrimp Sauce	7.0
Graham Crackers	7.1
Lobster, cooked	7.1
Milk, peptonized	7.1
Bird's Nest Soup	7.2
Tea	7.2
Tofu (Soybean Curd)	7.2
Wax Gourd Drink	7.2
Corn, frozen	7.3
Cheese, Camembert	7.4
Peanut Soup	7.5
Conch	7.5
Egg White	8.0

www.ingramcontent.com/pod-product-compliance
Lightning Source LLC
Chambersburg PA
CBHW031118020426
42333CB00012B/137